DEFINITION IS A DEFINITE HIT!

"Joyce has taken my time-tested principle 'the true pyramid system' and used it to invent THE MOST FAT-BURNING, TIME-EFFICIENT WORKOUT EVER!"
—**JOE WEIDER**, publisher of *Shape*,
Muscle and Fitness, and *Men's Fitness*

"SIMPLE INSTRUCTIONS—EASIER TO FOLLOW than any other similar book—and unique in its aerobic effect, while at the same time muscle-shaping and building power! GREAT JOB!"
—**BOB KENNEDY**, editor, *Musclemag International*,
Nassau County Council of Physical Fitness

"*DEFINITION* is the first and only book on the market that gives the exerciser a chance to work out either three days a week for thirty minutes, or six days a week for fifteen minutes, and still GET A FAT-FREE, WELL-SHAPED, TONED BODY—IN A MATTER OF WEEKS."
—**LUD SHUSTERICH**, world powerlifting record holder,
member of the All Time Greats Bodybuilding Hall of Fame

"I have used this workout myself to add definition to my body—I HAVE SEEN PATIENT AFTER PATIENT SCULPT AND SHAPE THEIR BODIES AND TURN FLAB INTO FIRM AFTER USING JOYCE'S LATEST PROGRAM, *DEFINITION*. As a doctor who treats many patients with weight problems, I find myself keeping a stack of Joyce's books on hand—to give to my patients."
—**JUDE BARBERA**, M.D., assistant clinical profesor of surgery,
Downstate Medical Center

"The American Chiropractic Association has made Joyce Vedral an honorary member because of her contribution to health and fitness—specifically, her wonderful workout books. I recommend Joyce's books to my patients regularly. Her latest, *DEFINITION*, PROVIDES A FAST-PACED, TOTAL-BODY WORKOUT THAT WILL SCULPT AND DEFINE THE BODY WITHOUT ADDING BULKY MUSCLE!"
—**JACK BARNATHAN**, doctor of chiropractic,
chairman, Nassau County Council of Physical Fitness

"*DEFINITION* IS EVERY WOMAN'S DREAM. FINALLY, THE SHAPE WITHOUT THE BULK—AND IN ONLY FIFTEEN MINUTES A DAY!"
—**BETTY WEIDER**, cofounder of *Shape* magazine,
author of *Better and Better*

DEFINITION

Shape Without Bulk in 15 Minutes a Day!

Joyce L. Vedral, Ph.D.

WARNER BOOKS

A Time Warner Company

A NOTE FROM THE PUBLISHER

The information herein is not intended to replace the services of trained health care professionals. You are advised to consult with your health care professional with regard to matters relating to your health, and in particular regarding matters which may require diagnosis or medical attention.

Warner Books, Inc., 1271 Avenue of the Americas, New York, NY 10020

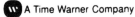 A Time Warner Company

Printed in the United States of America

ISBN 0-446-67069-3

Bodywear provided by Dance France (1-800-421-1543)
Photography by Don Banks
Hair and makeup by Jody Pollutro
Bathing suits by Nicole's Perfect Fit
Gym shoes by Reebok International
Cover design by Diane Luger
Cover photograph by Herman Estevez
Book design by Giorgetta Bell McRee

To you—my readers—by popular demand.
A book that lets you work your entire body
in one day if you choose to do so!

ACKNOWLEDGMENTS

To Joann Davis, for your continual support and enthusiasm.

Mel Berger, my agent, for your cheerful wisdom.

To Edna Farly, for your willingness to go the *extra, extra* mile in publicity!

To Grace Sullivan, for your indefatigable diligence.

To Diane Luger and Jacki Merri Meyer, for your dedication to the cover art.

To Larry Kirshbaum, Nanscy Neiman, and Emi Battaglia, for backing me up to the hilt.

To Don Banks, for your artistic photography.

To Jody Pollutro of Mélange of New York, for your talented hair and makeup.

To Dance France, for providing all the workout clothing—cover and interior.

To the Pritiken Longevity Centers in Miami and Los Angeles, for providing a place where physical and mental health are nurtured and restored.

To Ken's Fitness Center in Farmingdale, Long Island, for a wonderful gym—and they even have baby-sitting!

To David Bedwell and Family Fitness Centers throughout the United States, especially in Las Vegas, for an excellent all-around workout environment.

To the before-and-after women in this book—and to all of you who will soon become "afters."

To Judie Nixon, Debbie Stone, Amanda Moore, and Gloria Wise of La Costa Resort and Spa, for being up on the latest in fitness and providing a fun workout atmosphere.

To Nanette DiFalco and Stella of the Saks Fifth Avenue Club, for helping me to achieve "the look."

To Joe and Betty Weider—who started it all!

To family and friends, for your continual love and support.

To you, the women and men who have written to me requesting such a book. This one's for you!

CONTENTS

DEFINITION

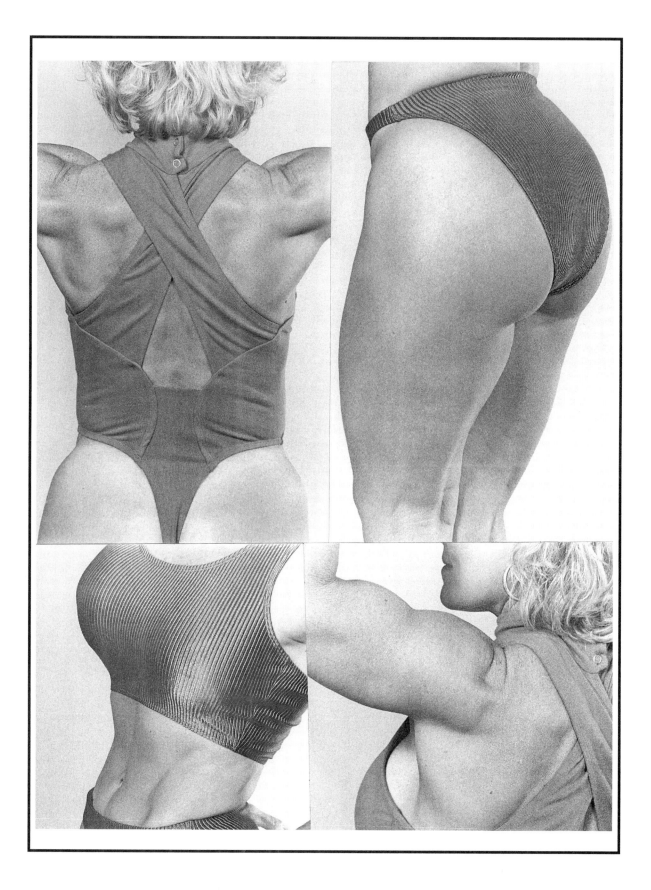

I

DEFINITION— SHAPE WITHOUT BULK IN FIFTEEN MINUTES A DAY

I don't want to put on size—I just want to be toned." "I'm busy. I don't have all day to spend working out." "I want a simple, no-nonsense workout." These are comments I hear a lot from people who don't want to get bulky muscles or to look even remotely like female bodybuilders—and who lead very busy lives. Well, there's great news. You *can* get toned without the bulk, and you can do this in minutes a day.

Yes. Amazingly, the two goals are completely compatible. Definition is a shorter workout that utilizes light weights in rapid succession and delivers definition—in shapely muscles—as opposed to the bulk that comes with a longer workout using heavier weights in slower succession. The fact is, in order to get maximum definition, *you must work very fast*, and indeed, you get a fat-burning aerobic workout while at the same time you achieve Definition.

Definition means the shaping and individualizing of your muscles by the delineation of your various muscle groups so that your entire body becomes tight, toned, symmetrical, and aesthetically beautiful. In short: your body becomes a delight to the eye and a joy to the touch.

THE RIGHT KIND OF MUSCLES

Not too long ago, women were reluctant to pick up a weight for fear that they would become huge and masculine-looking. Now, most women realize that it is not picking up a weight that will make them look like a hulking female body-builder, but how heavy that weight is, and what they do with that weight. Definition is carefully designed to suit your purposes to a T. It tells you what size weight to pick up, and exactly what to do with that weight, so as to achieve perfectly delineated feminine muscularity—yes, shape without the bulk. But how does this happen?

Remember back at grade school when you worked with a big lump of clay. At first the clay was an amorphous blob of material with no definite outline. But soon you began working with the clay and before you knew it, a specific figure was formed—and not by accident. It was your deliberate effort that shaped the clay into the desired form.

So it is with shaping your body. You can shape, form, define, and delineate your body by thoughtful effort—only you don't have to do the thinking. I have done it for you. Every movement in this workout is carefully designed and sequenced to sculpt your body into its most perfect form. It has taken years to perfect. If followed exactly as written, the results are guaranteed. You will have shape without bulk—clearly defined muscles under tight, smooth skin as opposed to soft, cellulite-ridden body parts—and you will do it in fifteen minutes a day, or thirty minutes every other day.

YOU WILL NEVER AGAIN BE TORTURED BY ENDLESS DIETING

It is sad to hear women talk about how they are still "fat," even though they have dieted down to even lower than their ideal weight. "What is wrong?" these women cry. Why is it that I'm never happy with my body, no matter how thin I am? Bev is an example of this (see page 31). In her before photograph she really didn't look that fat. In her after photo she was almost the same weight—but with muscle on her body this time, instead of fat—and look at the difference it made for her. She was able to get in shape without starving herself. She did the Definition workout and followed a reasonable, low-fat eating plan. And what's more, since building muscle raises your metabolism, Bev will burn more fat twenty-four hours a day—and can now eat more without getting fat!

YOU'RE NOT CRAZY—YOU *ARE* FAT—EVEN IF *THEY* DON'T SEE IT!

The truth is every woman needs to do a lot more working out, and a lot less dieting—because it is muscle that gives the body shape and form. Without muscles, you will always feel fat, because, guess what? You *are* fat. Your body is fat to the touch and fat to the sensation.

What am I saying—that you don't have to diet at all? No. If you are very much overweight, of course you will have to diet and lose some weight—but while you're losing it, you will be building an understructure of firm mini-muscles, so that once the excess fat is gone you will be left with a firm, sexy, well-defined body—not a skinny-fat body.

AS LONG AS YOU DON'T STOP WORKING OUT . . .

By following this workout, you will define and sculpt your body so that you will never again be obsessed with dieting, and even if you do decide to go wild and pig out for months at a time, and you gain weight from overeating, as long as you don't stop working out, you will still look a lot firmer and a lot sexier than you did when you were fat without the muscles under the fat.

One of my secrets for staying in shape is, I never stop working out. Because I know exactly how to lose the weight almost painlessly, and because I love food so much, I do allow myself to overeat and indeed sometimes pig out for weeks or months at a time. But because I don't stop working out, I never look like a regular "fat woman." Instead I look a little big and a little hefty. But the more important thing is, when I want to get back into shape, my job is really not that difficult. All I have to do is get sharp with my eating plan for a few months, continue working out, and I'm back in perfect shape.

But what would happen if I stopped working out and also pigged out at the same time? I would look flabby and round under the fat, and in the bargain, when I decided to get back in shape again, I would be depressed because I would have to reestablish the workout habit. My body would also feel so lethargic that I would probably have a real battle even starting to work out again. I would think, "Forget it. You're too far gone." It would be that much more difficult to get in shape.

DOES MUSCLE TURN TO FAT IF YOU STOP WORKING OUT?

No, no, no. Muscle does not turn to fat if you stop working out. What happens is, muscle slowly shrinks back to what it was before. If you also overeat, of course you gain fat while your muscles are shrinking. But the good news is, if you do stop working out, it takes just as long as you worked out to lose the muscles you gained, but only one third the time you worked out to get the muscles back. For example, if you worked out for a year and then stopped, it would take a year for you to lose all the muscles you had gained. But muscles have "memory." Once you started working out again, it would take only four months to regain the muscle that it took a year to gain the first time! So don't ever worry, "What if I stop working out, will it all turn to fat?" No. You have muscle memory in the bank, so to speak. It makes it that much easier for you to get in shape the next time.

THE BONES OF A TWENTY-FIVE YEAR OLD IN YOUR FIFTIES?

I've said it before. Working out with weights increases bone density—and in fact not only helps to prevent osteoporosis, but can reverse it! But until now I never knew exactly how dense my own bones were. Why? In general, I am not inclined to put myself on the table of a doctor's office and submit my body to any tests unless it is absolutely necessary. (Of course, I do get regular mammograms, pap tests, etc.) So why did I have my bone density tested now?

I had just passed the big "five oh" and was toying with the idea of going on hormone therapy—you know, estrogen replacement. My doctor informed me that I would be "insane" not to take it. But when I further questioned him, one of his strongest arguments was prevention of osteoporosis—or dangerous bone thinning that would cause hip fractures, etc., in later life. "But what if my bones are very dense to begin with?" I asked. "Well, they would have to be pretty thick! Don't assume your bones are thick," he said. I left thinking, "He's right. How do I know if I've never been tested?" So I decided to face the music and dance! I went to a radiologist and had what is called the QCT-Bone Mineral TM Analysis.

The results were so astounding that the radiologist called me at home the next day. "I've never seen anything like it," he said. "You went off the curve. Your bones are almost double the density of women in your age category— and more dense than an in-shape twenty-five-year-old. Everyone in the office was looking at your results in amazement. How do you do it?" I told him that I work out with weights the right way.

A few days later I got the written report. *My bone density is 219.3, whereas the lower average for women in my age category is 124!* And indeed my bones were more dense than women in excellent health—in their twenties.

What is the point of my telling you this? The best insurance policy against osteoporosis is to create solid, dense bones! I didn't touch a weight until I was approaching forty! I'll bet if I'd had my bones tested before that, they would have been much thinner. I can't go back and prove anything—but I can say that tests have been done on people in their eighties and nineties, who in a matter of months were able to increase their bone density to the point where they transformed themselves from being wheelchair-bound not only to walking, but to doing all kinds of things that they could never do again![1]

Note:

1. Interview with Dr. Sydney Bonnick, director, Osteoporosis Services, Cooper Clinic, Dallas, Texas, by John Stossel, ABC News, *20/20*, May 10, 1991, show #1119. New York: *Journal Graphics*, pp. 7–9.

YOU'RE THE BOSS—A WORKOUT THAT SUITS YOUR NEEDS

There are two pieces of good news for every woman who wants to get in shape but must fit her workout into her very busy schedule: 1) you can get in shape in only *fifteen minutes a day* (six days a week); or: 2) you can exercise your entire body in one workout day—and take the next day off—so that you only have to work out for *thirty minutes every other day* (three days a week). By doubling up, and working thirty minutes, you free yourself for other things on days when it may be inconvenient to work out. This is very important for most women.

THE STREAMLINED, POWER-PACKED WORKOUT

The Definition workout is more than revolutionary for those of you who know that in my previous books I have always recommended exercising one half of your body on workout day one, and the other half of your body on workout day two, and so on. How is it now possible to exercise the entire body in one workout day? The answer is simple. The Definition workout streamlines the exercises into *time-saving movements*, and utilizes a principle I've never used before in any of my books—the *true pyramid system*.

The following is an example of *the true pyramid system*, the method you will be using in this workout.

NEW SYSTEM: TRUE PYRAMID

Set 1: one-pound dumbbells—twelve repetitions
Set 2: two-pound dumbbells—ten repetitions
Set 3: three-pound dumbbells—eight repetitions
Set 4: two-pound dumbbells—ten repetitions
Set 5: one-pound dumbbells—twelve repetitions

You may be familiar with the old system, *the modified pyramid system*, presented in my other books. That system asked you to do only three sets per exercise—to rise in weights to the top of the pyramid, and then stop once you had used your heaviest weights. Here is a sample of that system.

OLD SYSTEM: MODIFIED PYRAMID

Set 1: one-pound dumbbells—twelve repetitions
Set 2: two-pound dumbbells—ten repetitions
Set 3: three-pound dumbbells—eight repetitions

Look up above and notice that the *new* system asks you to also *descend* the pyramid, adding two more sets by gradually reducing your weights until you arrive back at your beginning weights. These additional two sets make the difference between a modified and a true pyramid.

But what is the purpose of the additional two sets? By descending the pyramid, the muscle is coaxed to push itself just a little bit further—lured by the lighter weights, even though it may be tempted to quit. In this way, the muscle is challenged to the utmost degree. Maximum fat is burned and ultimate definition is realized, because more repetitions have been executed without resting.

But the benefit of the full pyramid system goes further than that. Because it requires the exerciser to perform those two additional sets, it eliminates the need for as many exercises as were previously required, and as a result cuts down workout time. In other words, by doing two exercises, you have performed ten sets (five sets each), whereas before you had to perform three exercises to get only nine sets (three sets each).

So what is the big deal about that, you might ask? In not having to change exercises, time is saved. There is both less thinking and less movement involved due to the limited need for repositioning for new exercises.

Finally, the Definition workout eliminates the time-consuming one-arm- or one-leg-at-a-time exercises (which double your workout time). The end result is either a much shorter daily workout (fifteen minutes) or the option of exercising your entire body in one day—combining two workouts in one, and freeing yourself on three days of the week (in addition to the regular off day) to do other things demanded by your very busy life.

WHY THE FIFTEEN-MINUTE WORKOUT IS EQUAL TO AN HOUR'S WORKOUT!

How can an effective workout be accomplished in only fifteen minutes a day? The simple answer is elimination of most rest periods—and shortening of the few rests that are allowed. Let's take a closer look. Most people who work out with weights rest an average of a minute between sets. Let's see how this affects workout time.

We'll use the example of a typical workout where the exerciser works one half of the body—four body parts—and does at least ten sets of various exercises for each of these body parts.

Okay. So we're talking about four times ten sets, or forty sets and forty possible rest periods of a minute each—that is forty minutes wasted resting. Definition allows no rests until you have completed ten sets (a full body part), and then allows only a fifteen-second rest—a total of four fifteen-second rests, or a minute rest. So with the Definition workout, you are resting one minute and saving thirty-nine minutes you would have wasted resting. And in the bargain, by not resting those thirty-nine minutes, you gain an aerobic effect and burn more fat.

Why then, you might ask, does anyone rest a minute between sets? They do it because they are probably lifting heavier weights, with the goal of adding significant muscle mass—in which case such rests are needed. But your goal is not to gain significant muscle mass—but rather to achieve petite, feminine muscularity with maximum definition.

So, how many minutes is your fifteen-minute workout really worth? Fifty-four minutes—or to round it off, almost an hour. See what I mean? You are packing into an intense fifteen minutes, a fifty-four-minute workout—and if you work the whole body in one workout day, you are packing into that thirty minutes 108 minutes, or nearly a two-hour workout. Not a bad bargain? And there is no catch, unless of course, the catch is, you cannot go as heavy as you would if you took more rests—and in turn, won't get as much muscle mass.

One final point. Because you are hardly resting, you build up a momentum—in a sense, you get on a roll. You don't have time to think after doing a few sets, "I think I'll stop. I'm tired" or "I'm bored." This workout really moves. You start it, and before you know it, it's over and you've accomplished the world—and in only fifteen minutes.

THE EXTRA MILE: WONDER WOMAN AND DRAGON LADY ROUTINES

But what about those of you who want to work longer than fifteen minutes a day—or longer than thirty minutes every other day? Perhaps you want to achieve a super-defined hard-as-a-rock razor-sharp body? You can take advantage of the Wonder Woman routine, which adds one exercise per body part, bringing your workout up to twenty-two minutes a day, or forty-four minutes every other day. Or you can really go for broke and do the Dragon Lady routine, which adds fourteen minutes a day—and you can work out either twenty-nine minutes a day or fifty-eight minutes every other day. But remember, no matter which workout you choose to do—the regular, the Wonder Woman, or the Dragon Lady—you are getting not double, not triple, but four times as much for your money (if time is money, and in my book, it is!).

HOW AND WHY I DISCOVERED THIS WORKOUT

Since the writing of my best-selling books, *The Fat-Burning Workout* and *Bottoms Up!,* I have received hundreds of letters from women asking me for a workout that would give them more definition and shape than ever, but one that was more convenient in two ways: a shorter workout, taking less time in a given day; and, more important, one that would give them the option of working the entire body in one day so that they could have the next day free to take care of other business.

Sure. I could have told them—no problem. Just double up and do the whole Fat-Burning Workout or Bottoms Up! workout in one day. But that would not have been fair, because I know that with these workouts the average, or even above average, person would become too exhausted if she tried to exercise her entire body in one session; and even if she could accomplish the workout, by the last third of the workout, she would become tired and begin to slack off—and body parts exercised toward the end of the workout would not be shaped and formed properly. In short, her body would look "half-baked," rather than fully developed—and I didn't want anyone walking around with a brand-name Joyce Vedral body looking half-baked. No way. I do have a reputation to consider.

So I continued experimenting, at first on myself, and later on other women—until I came up with a routine that could be achieved in a shorter period of time in daily sessions or would not exhaust the exerciser if doubled up, and into the bargain, would yield maximum definition and petite, feminine muscularity. Amazingly, the two goals were completely compatible—a shorter workout that yields more definition as opposed to a longer workout that yields more muscle size. The fact is, in order to get maximum definition, you must work very fast, and indeed you get an aerobic workout while at the same time achieving Definition.

MORE DEFINITION THAN EVER BEFORE: HOW THIS WORKOUT WORKS

This workout is based upon the threefold system of the true pyramid as explained above: the superset—doing two exercises for a body part in pairs, without resting; and the speed set—not taking rests until all exercises for a given body part are completed. (This simple method will be clearly explained in "How to Do the Definition Workout," Chapter 6, and reviewed in each exercise instruction.) The workout requires extremely light weights because of its intensity—you hardly rest at all. For this reason, even if you've been working with weights for quite some time, I prefer that you start with the bantam weight set of one-, two-, and three-pound dumbbells. (Those of you who have used one of my programs before may opt to go a little higher—see page 78 for guidelines.)

YOU CAN DO IT AT HOME OR AT WORK WITH LIGHT DUMBBELLS AND A BENCH OR "STEP"

One of the most wonderful things about this workout is you can practically do your workout anywhere—at home, at work, or even on the road. You can in fact switch on and off, doing your workout in the office when convenient (you can simply get a spare set of one-, two-, and three-pound dumbbells and keep them at work) and at home when you feel like it. And when you're on the road you can compromise and just take the one-pound dumbbells with you, and you'll be adding to your baggage weight a total of only two pounds. (The dumbbell weight is always calculated as each: when I say a set of ones, twos, and threes, I mean two one-pound dumbbells, two two-pound dumbbells, and two three-pound dumbbells.) You can get away with not using the other two sets of dumbbells while traveling by compensating with your own force—and using continual tension (see page 51). Another idea is to carry three-pound water weights (see page 257 to order).

For those of you who like to work out in a gym, of course you can do it. Only you will be using the free weights provided by the gym, rather than the machines. However, if you like the machines, note that I tell you under "Machines, etc." which machines can be used to replace the free weights.

But what about a bench? A bench is a good investment if you have the room for it, but if you don't, you can use a step. As you can see (pages 117–183) I use a step in place of a bench for my entire workout, and a chair when necessary.

WHY DEFINITION IS ALSO ALMOST PURE AEROBICS!

What is required for a workout to be considered aerobic? Technically speaking, an aerobic workout is a physical fitness activity that gets your pulse rate up to between 60 percent and 80 percent of its capacity, and causes it to stay there for twenty or more minutes. But now many fitness experts agree that even if you work for twelve to fifteen minutes, you still get the aerobic effect. In fact, many experts are recommending "aerobic spurts" even if they are as short as ten minutes.

There are almost no rests in the Definition workout—and the few rests that are taken are only seconds long—and are not long enough to allow the heart to slow down significantly.

WHAT ABOUT DIET?

If you are overweight you will want to follow the low-fat never-go-hungry eating plan provided in Chapter 9. In addition, if you want to strut your stuff for a special occasion, there is a special high-definition show-off emergency diet that you can follow for seven days.

In any case, the eating plan allows you to consume food as often as you choose—it gives you many unlimited anytime night or day selections, three square meals, and two hearty snacks! And what's more, you don't have to get involved in fancy cooking or elaborate meal planning. Just follow the guidelines in Chapter 9.

If you are not overweight, but are a skinny-fat (your body feels soft and mushy as opposed to firm and toned), you can continue to eat the way you do—however, take a look at the nutritional low-fat eating plan. It is a good idea for everyone to lower fat intake for health reasons. See page 208 for further discussion on this subject.

WHO CAN DO THIS WORKOUT?

This workout is for the following: 1) Newcomers who have never worked out a day in their lives. You will be using the one-, two-, and three-pound dumbbells, and one of the break-in plans on pages 81–84. 2) Old hands—people who have been working out for years and experimenting with other workouts contained in books I've written, or people who are serious bodybuilders and want to burn maximum fat and achieve more definition. 3) People who are intermediates—those of you who have dabbled in working out from time to time, and who are now ready to try a new, shorter, more power-packed workout.

You can do this workout if you are a skinny-fat, if you are only ten to fifteen pounds overweight, or if you are a *hundred pounds overweight.* (Don't worry. The workout won't cause heavy people to look even bigger. The mini-muscles being formed under the fat will not put on size. I promise!)

In short, no matter how fat or thin you are, no matter where you are in your workout history, this workout can be for you.

But *what about men?* Yes. Men can do this workout, but men have the lucky break of being able to leave out the hip-buttocks exercises, because men do not have childbearing hips. Most men, of course, will be able to double the weight of most women because of their strength and muscle size. Men should follow the same guidelines as women as to deciding on a beginning weight and adding weight to the routine as they get stronger (see page 78). Another idea for men is to go directly to my books addressed to them: *Top Shape* and *Gut Busters.*

For whom is this workout *not* suitable? People who want to put on significant size. Although I do provide an alternative way of using this workout to put on a little more muscle mass (see page 85), those of you who want to put on significant muscle mass should switch to my book *Now or Never* (see Bibliography), and follow the home or gym workout contained in that book.

What about age? With your doctor's permission of course, you can do this workout whether you are sixteen or sixty. In fact, you can do this workout if you are as young as thirteen, or if you're pushing ninety! Of course, no matter who you are, you must always check with your doctor before starting any training program.

IMPROVED EXERCISE INSTRUCTIONS AND TEAR-OUT WALL CHART

Due to popular demand, I have made a big improvement in the exercise instructions. I've added a section on sets, repetitions, and weights that tells you exactly which exercise you are supersetting with which exercise, how many reps to do of each, and how much weight to use. In addition, I include on pages 191–201 tear-out pages of the exercises paired exactly as you will do them (in reduced size so that they fit into a chart formation). You put these pages up on your wall for a handy chart—but of course I will assume that you have carefully read the exercise instructions first. The chart is for later convenience—so you won't have to keep referring back to the book.

BONUS ADVANTAGES OF THIS WORKOUT

I would be remiss if I did not at least brush upon the other wonderful side effects of this workout: added muscularity that raises your metabolism and allows you to eat more without getting fat; reversal of the aging process through replacing and adding muscle density and bone density; prevention and reversal of osteoporosis; added strength; improved posture; improved ability in sports; lowered cholesterol levels; lowered blood pressure; and for many, relief of chronic lower back, neck, and shoulder pain as a result of now achieving balanced musculature, strengthened muscles, and thickened bones—all of this in addition to tightening and toning the body and reshaping it into its most perfect form.

QUICK LIST—THE CHANGES YOU WILL SEE IN TWENTY-ONE DAYS!

- Definition of muscles in chest, shoulders, back, biceps, and triceps.
- Reduced dress or pants size.
- Increased metabolism so that you burn more fat during the day.
- Increased energy and strength.
- Improved posture.
- The sensation of being tighter and more toned—even in body parts that are not yet showing visible results.

LONG LIST—WHAT YOU WILL SEE IN TWENTY WEEKS

- The loss of between twenty-five and forty pounds of fat.
- The placement of firm, petite, defined muscles all over your body—muscles that take up less space than fat.
- A drop in dress or pants size by three or four sizes.
- The ability to eat and weigh more than previously without looking fat, and in fact, looking thinner than you did at a higher weight.
- The establishment of the workout habit—so that you no longer struggle with the idea of working out, but rather do it automatically.
- A rosier outlook on life due to increased self-esteem.
- Gradual increasing of bone density at any age.

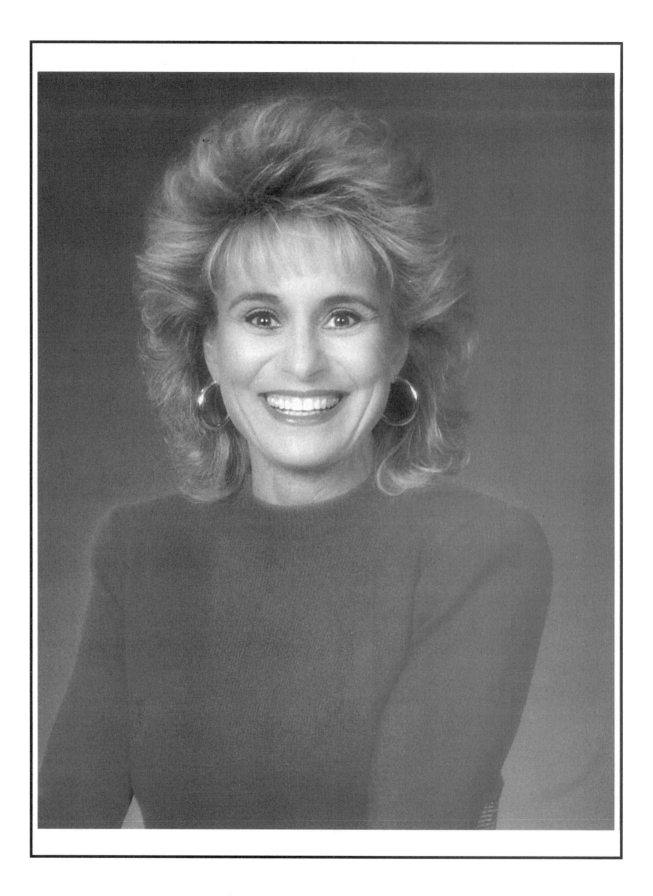

2

IF I CAN DO IT, YOU CAN DO IT TOO— MY STORY

At twenty-two years old, I was a petite ninety-eight pounds. Since I'm only five feet tall, that was a good weight for me. But I didn't stay that way. One year later, I weighed 108 pounds. A year later, I weighed 118 pounds. The next year the scale tipped 131. I remembered the words of my family and friends at my engagement party: "Enjoy that youthful figure, because once you get married, it all goes." And looking at those who were speaking to me, it appeared to be true: my mother, who was at the time about sixty pounds overweight; my aunt, who was over a hundred pounds overweight; and my cousin's wife, who was carrying a load of about forty extra pounds.

"It won't happen to me," I thought, because I had always been underweight. In fact, I remembered how at ten years old I hated the malteds (similar to milkshakes), and the Laquofort powder (a high-calorie weight-gain compound recommended by the family doctor). I was told that I had to force myself to down these drinks if I ever expected to gain weight. By the time I got to high school I was still skinny. I wished I had a shape like other girls. That's why it was so hard for me to believe that I had joined the fat group after three years of marriage—going from a size three to a thirteen—and the thirteens were getting tighter. What? Would I end up having to go to the "misses" department, like my mother?

It was small comfort to me that my sister was also getting fat. *She* was never underweight! I tried to rationalize the situation. "Oh, who cares," I thought. "Why do I have to be in shape? I was never a potential Miss America candidate in the first place. I'll never win a beauty prize, and anyway, I've already got my man." But switching gears, I took a then-radical women's lib point of view. "Why is it okay for men to get fat but not women? Why is it—thirty pounds overweight he's still sexy, but if a woman does it she's matronly?" Finally, I tried to adopt a philosophical stance. "So what if I'm fat. The mind is what's important, not the body—what you do to help people is more important than the way you look." I even went so far as to dig up a Bible verse: "For bodily exercise profiteth little."

But none of it worked. I became obsessed with my weight. When I would overhear comments from my students (I was a high school teacher at the time) such as, "Is she pregnant?" I would die a little more inside. My creativity was being drained, as much of my time and energy was diverted to the issue of my weight. In spite of myself much of my time was taken up with conversations about the latest miracle diet.

I almost died when one day a student seeing me from afar mistakenly called me Mrs. Stack, a teacher who wore the same hairstyle as I did, only who was much older than I, and who I thought looked fat and matronly. I began to dread holidays where I would see people I had not seen for some time, dreading the inevitable remark: "Wow, did you gain weight. What happened?" Ever on the alert for a comment about my increasing girth, I armed myself with defensive repartee: "I'm just bloated, it's that time of the month," or "No I didn't. It's just the dress."

Finding something to wear became more and more trouble. Tired of buying bigger and bigger sizes, I sidestepped the problem by dredging up the dressmaking skills I had learned in junior high. I began making my own clothing and selecting patterns that would hide my shape—tentlike dresses—the "A-line." Here I was, only in my twenties, and already I was looking for ways to obscure my body.

The final blow came when after a physical required by my job, the doctor looked down at my protruding stomach and said, "For such a young woman, you've really let yourself go." Rendered speechless by the desire to cry, I barely managed to get out of the office. Then my embarrassment turned to rage. First against the doctor, whose face I had wanted to slap, and then at myself—stuffing myself so full that evening that I could hardly move from the chair to the bed. I still remember how that night as I lay in bed I felt so out of control—so alone, and how I drifted off to sleep thinking of a woman in our church who was now a shut-in because she had gained over four hundred pounds—and now people from the church had to bring her food.

That's when I began my search for a diet that would once and for all do the job for me. My first stop was Weight Watchers. And watch weight I did. In fact, I became so obsessed with watching my weight that when I knew I didn't lose weight that week, I would try to cheat the scale by taking laxatives and diuretics the night before weigh-in day, in spite of warnings from my Weight Watchers lecturer never to do this!

I managed to follow this diet plan to the T, weighing and measuring everything I ate, constantly thinking about portion allotments of food ("Lord have mercy," I thought. "Is this the way I'll have to live the rest of my life?"). Eventually I did lose weight. I got down to 103 pounds. Yet something was wrong. Now in my thirties, I noticed that my body was not as firm as it used to be in my early twenties—but instead was soft to the touch. I didn't have the shape I had dreamed I would have after losing the weight. In short, I had become a skinny-fat. To make matters worse, I quickly regained all the weight I had lost—and then some.

Since dieting alone had obviously not done the job, I began my search for an exercise plan that would give me back my shape. "I don't care if I have to work out five hours a day," I thought. *"I won't be fat."*

I took up the sport of judo. After sustaining a knee injury I was told to use the leg extension machine for rehabilitation. I found myself in a popular health spa where the trainers wore high heels and looked as if they were Playboy Bunnies. Wanting more than a healthy knee, I listened attentively to their fitness advice (there was a different trainer each week—these women didn't stay at the job for too long, it seemed). I still remember how sad I felt when the young sexy twenty-something trainer said to me, as she looked at me with pity, "You can't do much at your age, but if you follow this workout it will help to reshape your thighs" (she showed me a tedious, ineffective floor-work regimen).

As time went by, I was given at least fifteen different programs, including circuit training, but after a couple of years of working out for two hours a day, six days a week, my body did not show any clear improvement. All I had to show for my effort was a very slight improvement of my muscle tone and strength—but absolutely no change to my basic shape, and a dreadful rapidly aging body with cellulite that was invading new territory every time I dared to scrutinize my body in the mirror.

Then I got lucky. One day a bodybuilder approached me. He said, "I see you here every day. You work very hard, but you're doing it all wrong. *It's not how much you do but what you do that counts.* You would get better results by working out the right way for only thirty minutes a day—and you'd see results in only a few months." He invited me to try the bodybuilding principles he had learned from Joe Weider. I started to protest, thinking, "Sure. I couldn't get in shape in two hours a day for two years, and this man is telling me I can get in shape in a few months in a shorter daily workout." But just as I was ready to open my mouth I looked up at the man and observed his perfectly symmetrical, hard, muscular body. A lightbulb went on as I thought to myself, *"Hello! Are you intelligent, Joyce? Look at the man's body.* This man has spent his life learning the secrets of getting in shape. His body is the proof of it. Why are you arguing with him? He must know what he's talking about."

So I listened. But I did more than that. I landed a freelance job writing for *Muscle and Fitness* magazine, where I was able to learn the basics of body shaping by interviewing Joe Weider, the owner of the magazine, and the champion bodybuilders featured in the magazine. I devised a workout that utilized the basic principles of bodybuilders but with lighter weights and less workout time, and just as the bodybuilder had suggested, in a matter of months my body was significantly reshaped. For the first time in my life, my thighs were beginning to have definition. I could see a quadriceps muscle clearly forming, and the skin that was hanging over my knee was now firm—held taut against the shapely thigh muscle. My previously skinny arms and sloping shoulders now had sexy curves, and my protruding lower abdomen was beginning to flatten, while my upper abdominals showed definition. Even my upper back looked pretty. I never knew I had muscles there—but now I knew because I could see the clear delineation.

I also learned the secrets of proper eating. By interviewing scores of body-builders, I found out that it's not how much you eat but what you eat that counts. For the first time in my life I was able to eat not only three square meals a day, but two hearty snacks and a variety of free unlimited complex carbohydrates all day long whenever I was hungry. I learned, years before the medical community came out strong against a high-fat diet, that fat was the real enemy when it comes to weight loss—not food in general. I found myself no longer obsessing about food because, finally, food was no longer the issue.

In three months all of my friends were asking for my secrets. I ended up spending an awful lot of time writing down my routine. I even coached three of my friends—and had before-and-after photos of their progress. Frustrated, and wanting to be relieved of the task of personal training, I went to bookstores in search of a book I could recommend to these women, but low and behold, the only books available were hard-core male and female bodybuilding books that would make women look like Arnold, or ones with the silly, ineffective routines typically given to women. So I continued to work for free—writing down the routine I had invented with the knowledge I had acquired about bodybuilding techniques.

Soon I became a self-appointed teacher, imposing myself on women who I noticed were doing ineffective workouts. "Hey, you're wasting your time in the gym," I would say. "I used to do that. It will never get you in shape." But most of the women, after glancing at my now shapely, muscular body, resented my unsolicited advice. "She was born that way," I heard one woman say. "She probably spends all her time here," the other responded. In any case, I realized that I was going to have to find a more effective way to get my message across. Being a Ph.D. in English literature and a published author of parent-teen books, I had already established myself as a writer, so I asked my agent to approach a publisher about a book containing my techniques.

I'll never forget my first interview with Warner Books. Armed with the before-and-after photographs of the women, and a before photo of myself, I sat in the office wearing a conservative business suit explaining why my workout was different from any other offered to women who wanted to get into shape but did not want to look like a bodybuilder. I talked and talked, but as I looked around, I noticed that my listeners were only mildly interested, occasionally yawning and looking at their watches. Then, impulsively, I took off my jacket, stood up, and pulled up my blouse about five inches until my entire upper abdominal region was showing. I flexed my muscles and beat on my well-defined stomach and said, "Feel my abs."

The whole atmosphere in the room changed. Some were amused. Others were slightly embarrassed, but I had their attention. Quite taken aback, the men refused to take me up on my offer, but I managed to convince a few of the women to touch my stomach. They were quite impressed. "Hard as a rock," they said. "Did you ever have children?" (Yes I had.) "How did you do it?" In a few minutes I was flexing my arms, showing off my defined shoulders, and pointing to my no-longer-waving triceps. I even pulled up my skirt to show off my now shapely, cellulite-free thighs. The final straw was when I whipped out the before photograph of myself and the before-and-after photos of the three women I had put on the program. Before you knew it, it was a deal. My fitness-book-writing career had begun.

YOU ARE NOT ALONE—I'VE BEEN DOWN THAT ROAD

I had searched for over ten years for a way to lose weight and get in shape. During that time my scale weight went up and down and my body got softer and softer and fatter. Because of occasional starvation dieting, my body composition had changed and I lost muscle (the body literally eats itself when being starved). Even though I had stopped starvation dieting, the muscle I had lost never came back, because at the time, I didn't know the first thing about muscle building.

I know how it feels to be frustrated—to have been jerked around by every latest fad diet or miracle-cure exercise device. I once spent my hard-earned money on a Thighmaster type of device, only to leave it in the closet for years, and eventually throwing it out. I know how it feels to believe in your secret heart that the problem is really you—that in your case, there is no hope. You are just a pig with bad genetics and poor discipline, and you are doomed to a life of matronly misery. Because I know this, I can never rest until I have reached every woman who feels the way I used to feel—until I give each of you the secret that will allow you, once and for all, to get your body in shape, and get your weight under control so that you can go on with your life and devote your energy to more important things.

GET IT OUT OF THE WAY AND GET ON WITH YOUR LIFE!

After all, should most of your time be devoted to how you look? Of course not! But it will be unless you deal with the problem, because being fat and out of shape affects the way you feel physically and mentally. If you are fat and out of shape, your body is usually tired and lethargic and your mind is not alert. You are also frequently depressed. You're not as creative in whatever you are doing at the moment, whether it's writing a letter to a friend, figuring out a business problem, or dealing with family matters. So there's really little choice in the matter. It's time to get in shape so that you can clear the path for living up to your full potential.

If you are a teacher, you will be a better teacher if your mental energy is not being diverted by such thoughts as, "Did that student just say I look pregnant?"

If you are a sales rep, you will be more effective in your job if you are not always worrying about which outfit best hides your fat. No matter what you are in life—a doctor, a lawyer, or a full-time housewife and mother—you'll be a happier, more creative person if your energy is not being continually drained by preoccupation with negative thoughts about your body.

People see my body and they ask: "Is working out your life?" The answer is no. Absolutely not. Working out is a very small part of my life—but that very small investment of time sets me free to have a life because now I don't have to think about my body! It's in control. I can be creative and more effective in whatever life has to offer.

Get in shape. Get it out of the way. Get your mental energy back on track—where it should be. Allow yourself to fulfill the purpose for which you were born. Once and for all, end the slow, subtle theft of your vitality, your youth, and your very life.

WHY WOMEN GET FAT: MY STORY—YOUR STORY

You've heard my story. You know why I got fat and out of shape. Your story may be similar, but then again, it may be different. Like me, you may have a genetic proclivity toward bigness (everyone in my Russian family is or was overweight—as I often say on television, they look like boxes on wheels).

Perhaps you've gotten fat out of loneliness. Maybe you don't feel that you're getting the love you deserve, so you eat with two forks to fill the gaping hole in the center of your being. Perhaps you eat out of frustration: every time you get some aggravation—on the job, from your boyfriend or husband, from the children—you eat. "I'll soothe myself," you think. "At least I can enjoy this food," you say.

Or you may have gained the weight because of pregnancy. You really let yourself go at that time, thinking, "Finally no one can see my shape anyway, I might as well eat," or reasoning, "If I can't eat now, when can I eat—after all, I do have to think of the health of the baby," or believing, "Oh, I don't have to worry. It will all come off after the baby is born." Or maybe you tried your best not to gain too much weight when you were pregnant, but in spite of your efforts, you did anyway.

Maybe your reason for gaining weight is not frustration, but contentment. Perhaps you got married and settled down to the good life. You and your husband enjoy going out to dinner and you enjoy cooking and having company over. Before you know it, you're getting fatter and fatter. In such a case, perhaps when you try to lose weight, you find that your husband is not supportive. And in fact, a well-meaning man can sabotage your efforts. Content with the status quo, he brings you home goodies that are too tempting to resist.

Your husband, however, may not be so well-meaning. Maybe he feels more secure keeping you fat. After all, if you lose weight he will have to deal with men looking at you—and in his deeper self, he may be afraid of losing you. In any case, your efforts to lose weight are hindered by him because every time you start to lose weight he either complains that you're not cooking for him anymore, he brings home goodies, or he criticizes you, saying you looked better the other way.

Perhaps you have gotten fat because you're bored with your life. Your life is humdrum and nothing really excites you. You end up spending a lot of time sitting in front of the TV and eating.

Maybe you gained weight because you have somewhere along the line lost your "self" to your husband and/or your children. You got married and, without realizing it, you slowly sacrificed your goals and your dreams to the family. Now your only purpose is to be a good wife and mother. Without realizing it, "you" disappeared. You honestly didn't see that you were getting fatter and fatter. But on those days when the core of your being, that part of the self that can never be erased, calls out, "Help, help. I'm drowning," you realize that you are not happy this way.

Maybe you got fat because you believed that getting fat and out of shape is the inevitable result of getting older. After all, everyone knows that every year after thirty, muscle begins to atrophy at the rate of up to half a pound a year, and when that happens, metabolism naturally slows down. Why, of course, everyone gets fatter with age. Even eating the same amount of food that you consumed in your twenties will cause weight gain in your forties because of muscle loss. And then when you take into account that you are naturally less active in your forties than you were in your twenties, and are using up less calories, getting fat is the most natural thing in the world.

Perhaps you didn't really gain weight at all—you just seemed to lose your shape as the years went by. You're not a big eater to begin with, and/or you have a high metabolism, but as the years went by, and as your muscles began to slowly atrophy, you became a skinny-fat. Or you may be a young woman whose muscles did not yet begin to atrophy. Yet you are not satisfied with your shape, and many parts of your body feel fat, so in some ways you think of yourself as a skinny-fat. You think, "Oh well, I guess it's just my genetics. I'm doomed to this body for life."

IT DOESN'T HAVE TO BE THAT WAY

But it doesn't have to be that way. Not at all. You can reshape your body and get the body you never had. You can actually improve your "genetics"—what you were given by nature—by placing petite, sexy muscles in all the right places. If you are a skinny-fat who has lost muscle tone due to aging, you can regain the lost muscle by working out. You can not only replace what you lost but add more, so that you can look sexier and eat more than before without getting fat.

If you've gotten fat and out of shape because of loss of self, you can regain the self you lost by doing something for yourself—by deciding to work out and create the body of your dreams. Once you begin to see your body changing as a result of your own daily actions, you'll regain the sense of self you lost along the way. One thing will lead to another and you'll begin to rebuild your life in other areas too.

If you gained weight out of boredom, once you begin working out, your energy level will come up and your self-esteem will rise. You'll find yourself thinking about taking a course in evening school, joining a dance group, or taking up self-defense. All kinds of exciting ideas will occur to you.

If your reason for getting fat was a sabotaging husband, you can ask him to join you in your workout. Two of the men in my fitness book *Top Shape* did just that! If he's not interested, you can still get in shape, and once he sees that you don't try to pressure him to change, and you don't leave him for another man just because you are in shape, and how much sexier you are to him now, perhaps he'll even begin to encourage you in your efforts.

If you got fat because of contentment, you can motivate yourself to get in shape to regain the peace of mind you've now lost. If your weight gain was due to pregnancy, realize that like Dana, after you deliver the baby, you don't have to carry around a "fat baby"—the excess weight gain—for the rest of your life. You can decide to "deliver" that other baby, once and for all, and it may not take nine months. Dana did it in 12 weeks! (Read her story on page 28).

Finally, if you put on the pounds out of loneliness or feeling a lack of love, you can shape up by giving yourself love and attention. With every movement of the dumbbell you will feel self-love developing, and with every sign of well-defined feminine muscularity on your body, you will want to kiss your hand and say, "I love you. You're the greatest." The self-empowerment you feel will emanate from your being and you'll find yourself attracting and talking to more people. You'll begin to make friends of both sexes, and you'll become motivated to pursue goals and even dreams.

WE'RE DIFFERENT, YET THE SAME: THE COMMON DENOMINATOR

The underlying reason for getting out of shape is the same for all of us: neglect. Even a car would begin to look shoddy and would eventually stop running if we refused to give it at least the minimum care. Yet we blissfully neglect to care for our muscles properly, and we refuse to feed our bodies with healthy foods. We can change all of this by doing something different. *The definition of insanity is to do the same thing and to expect something different to happen.* It's time to stop doing the same thing you've been doing. It's time to give your body the attention it needs and so well deserves so that you can get it in shape once and for all, and free your energy for the important things you want to do in life.

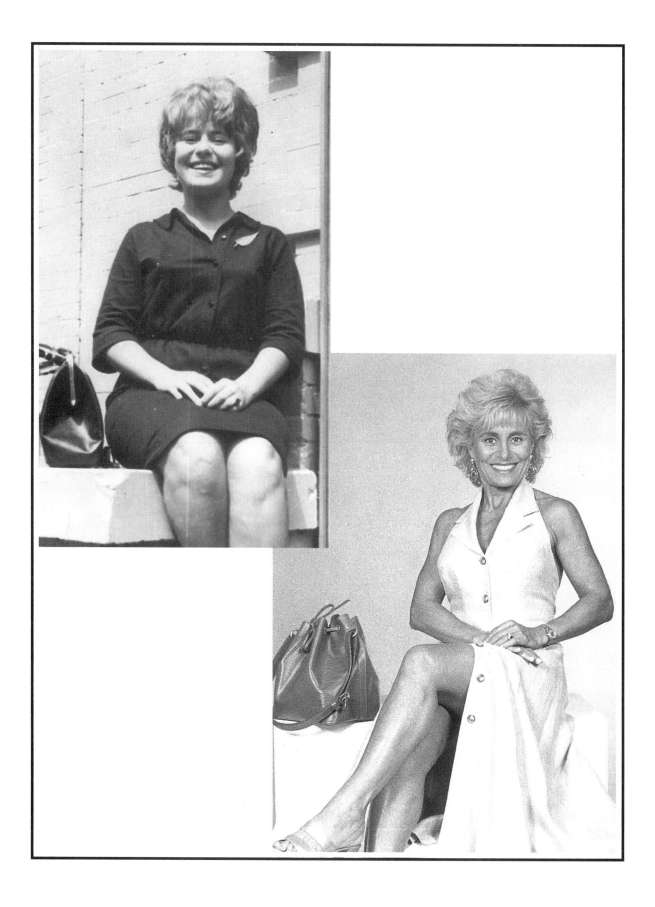

3

BEFORE AND AFTER

JOYCE VEDRAL, AGE FIFTY-TWO—
FROM SIZE THIRTEEN TO SIZE FIVE

As the saying goes, a picture is worth a thousand words. Look at me when I was a month short of twenty-six sitting on the church steps—and look at me now at fifty-two, double that age. As I mentioned in Chapter 2, I began gaining weight the moment I got married, at which time I went from ninety-eight pounds, a size three, to 131 pounds, a size thirteen pushing fifteen! I remember how I started tearing up all my "fat photographs." I now wish I had saved some of those family picnic photos when I was even fatter—and in a bathing suit. But I think you can get the idea if you take a look at my hips.

I am of course thrilled with the results I've gotten with the workout. But frankly, I'm even more impressed with you, the women who read my books and get in shape by following the instructions and the photographs. In this chapter you'll find those women—women who, just like you will do, took action and got results. They had no personal help from me. They did not use a video. They had the exact same instructions that you do—only before this book was published—and just look at them now, as you compare them to their before pictures. At the end of this chapter I provide a space for your own before-and-after photograph, and if you send it to me, after we talk, if you wish, you may end up in a future book.

BARBARA, FIFTY-THREE YEARS OLD— FROM SIZE FOURTEEN TO SIZE TEN IN TEN WEEKS!

Barbara is the mother of three children aged fifteen, twenty-five, and twenty-seven. She's very active in community affairs, and helps her husband run his real-estate and camera store businesses.

You may recognize Barbara from my first book, *Now or Never.* She had gotten herself into shape by working out for ninety minutes a day with that workout, but then her oldest son got cancer, and with the constant trips to the hospital she was unable to find the time or the will to work out. Soon she stopped working out and began taking out her anxiety on eating. The more she ate, the fatter she got! Thankfully, her son was miraculously cured of cancer. ("Our church had twenty-four-hour prayer chains going," she says.)

Barbara had just about given up getting in shape again. "I don't have it in me anymore to work out—not even for an hour a day. Call it old, call it not motivated, call it whatever you want. I'm just not doing it. I guess it's too late for me." But when I showed Barbara this new workout plan, and told her that she could either work out for only fifteen minutes six days a week, or for thirty minutes three days a week, she said, "I can do that. I'll give it a try. What have I got to lose?"

She did, and look what happened to Barbara in only ten weeks. She went from a size fourteen to a size ten, lost eighteen pounds, and reshaped her entire body. "I still have a way to go," says Barbara. "I want to go down at least one more size—and I know the last ten pounds are going to take longer, so I'm going to be patient, but I can tell you one thing, this is more than a weight loss program. Before, even if I went on diets and lost weight, I was still flabby and I felt fat. Now I feel firm and I'm not ashamed of my body. At first I couldn't believe that you could do this in only fifteen minutes a day—but it did work. I guess because you're not trying to put on sizeable muscle."

P.S. Barbara is my sister!

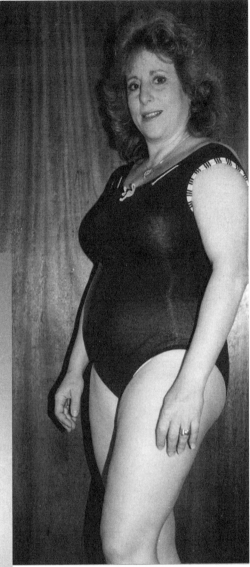

Barbara, 53, before, size 14

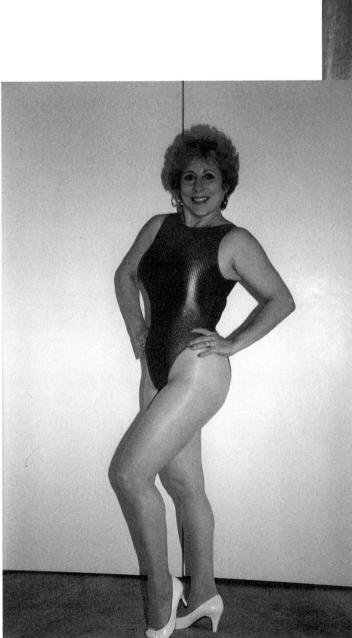

Barbara after ten weeks, size 10

DANA, TWENTY-FOUR YEARS OLD— FROM A SIZE THIRTEEN AFTER-PREGNANCY WEIGHT TO A SIZE FOUR IN FOURTEEN WEEKS!

Dana weighed 164 pounds just before she gave birth. "I had to stay in bed because of complications and that really put on the weight. But I was hoping against hope that I would lose most of the weight after delivering." Dana was sadly disappointed to find that she only lost ten pounds and weighed a hefty 154, and was now a size thirteen. (Before getting pregnant she was a size eleven.) Dana did the workout, and in a matter of weeks Dana said, "I could see a huge difference—for the first time in my life, I could actually see and feel muscles on my body instead of flab."

In fourteen weeks, Dana went down to 120 pounds—a weight loss of thirty-four pounds. Some of that weight loss was obviously additional after-birth water loss. But it's not the weight loss that impresses me. It's the change in the shape and definition of her body—and the resulting change in her dress size! "I have tried many exercise programs in the past," says Dana. "None of them brought the quick results that your workout brought. Best of all, I've finally gotten a chance to do what I've always wanted to do but couldn't. I'm a model now for a few agencies in Atlanta, and I'm loving every minute of it!"

Dana, 24, nine months pregnant

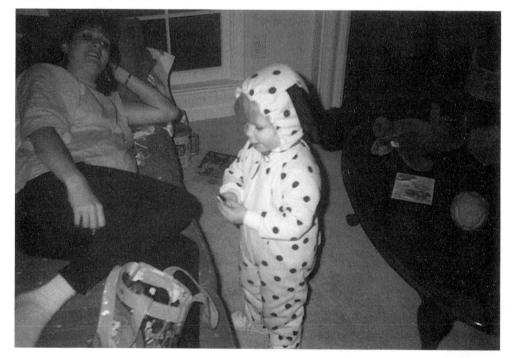

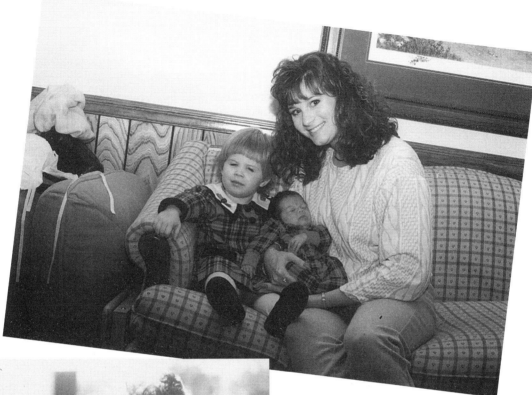

Dana right after delivery, size 13

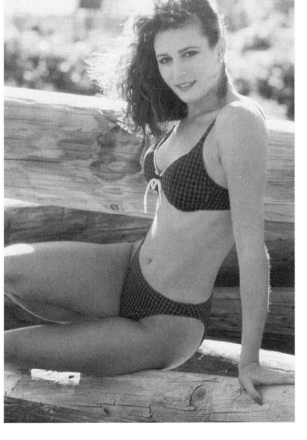

Dana after fourteen weeks, size 4

BEV, FIFTY YEARS OLD—FROM SIZE TWELVE TO SIZE SIX IN TWELVE WEEKS

Bev is a busy woman with three children ranging from nineteen to twenty-seven! She lives on a small farm with her husband—and there's plenty of work to be done. In addition, says Bev, "I work full time in an office at a high school, so my job is fairly sedentary." At first Bev didn't think she would have the time or the discipline to follow through on the workout. But after seeing how easy it was, and how much better she felt after the workout, she made a daily plan and stuck to it using the six-day-a-week plan. "I love the workout because it gives me a total-body workout and an aerobic workout too."

After twelve weeks look what Bev was able to do. "I feel totally good about my body now—and stronger, more fit and muscular than before I had my three girls. My daughters are proud of their mother and my husband is thrilled."

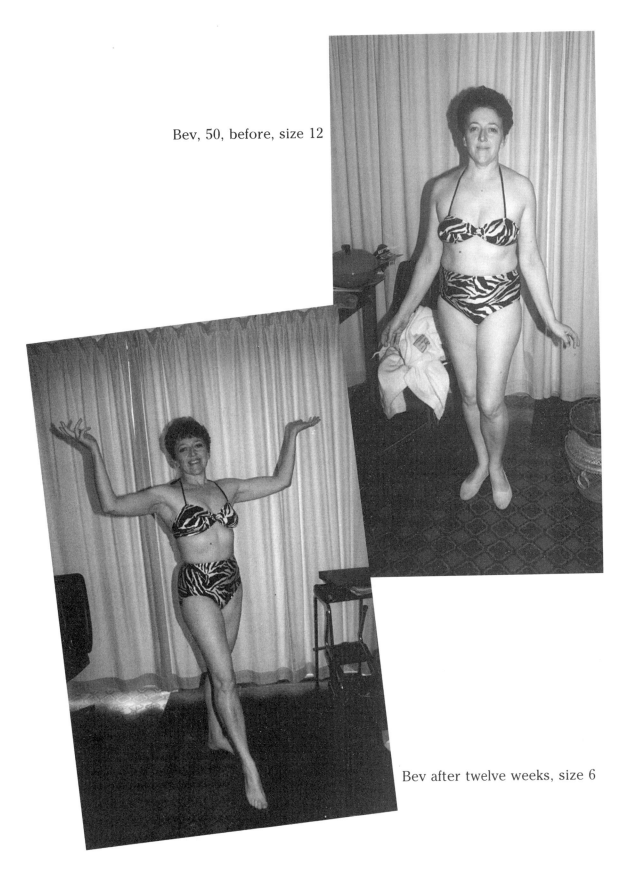

Bev, 50, before, size 12

Bev after twelve weeks, size 6

DEBBIE, THIRTY-ONE YEARS OLD—FROM SIZE SIXTEEN TO SIZE SEVEN IN TWENTY WEEKS!

Debbie is a nurse's aid. She was so fat that she tore up most of her before photographs. She had to call all of her relatives until finally she was able to come up with this one fat photograph that shows only her leg. When Debbie started this workout she didn't expect much to happen—but she thought she would give it a try. To her amazement, once she started the workout her body began to make dramatic changes. "Everything started going north," she says. "The fat began to melt and the muscles began to pop. This workout has made me so strong I can now lift my patients into bed—before I had to call another aid to help me. And now, at least I have a waist for them to grab me. Before they had to hold on to those love handles. I also have so much more energy all day long.

"What do I love most about this program—the way it shaped and defined my legs, my stomach, my arms, my whole body? Yes. I love all of that, but the body part that has been most affected by this workout is my mind. Now I'm confident, and I know I don't have to sell myself short."

Debbie lost forty pounds in all—most of it fat, some of it water! Once again, it's not the weight loss that impresses me the most but the reshaping and defining of not only her body but her mind.

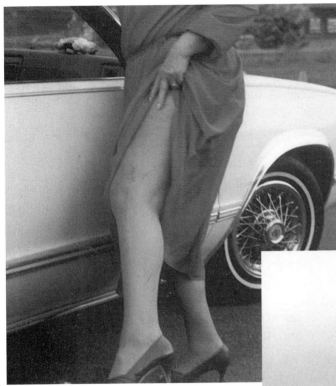

Debbie, 31, before, size 16

Debbie after twenty weeks, size 7

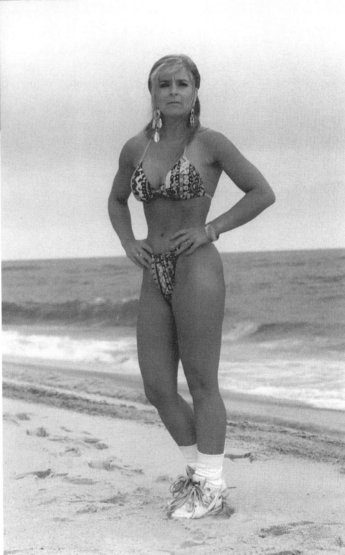

YOU WILL BE AN "AFTER" TOO!

If they can do it, you can do it too. I want you to take a before photo right now. Put on either a bathing suit, underwear, or tight-fitting clothing. Take the photograph against a noncluttered background. Hide the photograph somewhere and take another photograph wearing the same outfit in five weeks, another in ten weeks, another in fifteen weeks, and another in twenty weeks—five photographs in all. Watch your body's gradual metamorphosis from fat and flabby to lean, muscular, shapely, and defined. Send me the before and twenty-week photograph. I'd love to have you go on a television show with me, or perhaps be featured in a magazine article or a "fitness hall of fame" I'm planning to include in a future book. See page 257 for P.O. Box. Be sure to include a stamped, self-addressed envelope for a reply.

But don't stop taking photographs yet. If you can look this great in twenty weeks, wait until you see how your body continues to improve as time goes by—forty weeks, a year, two years. You just keep getting better and better as your muscles become more seasoned, and as you switch from time to time to one of my other workouts for variety and perfection (see Chapter 10 for a discussion of this).

Before Photograph   **After Twenty Weeks**

WHAT YOU WILL SEE AND FEEL WEEK BY WEEK

Week 1: You will feel sore but very proud.

Week 2: You will feel some soreness and begin to feel stronger.

Week 3: You will see traces of definition on your shoulders, biceps, and upper back.

Week 4: You will notice greatly increased energy. You'll start to see definition on your side and upper abdominal area and increasing cleavage in your breasts.

Week 5: The scale will have gone up and down, but by now your weight will have shifted—you've lost fat and gained muscle. Your body shape is changing subtly—you can see it in the mirror.

Week 6: You will notice more and more definition on your entire upper body. You continue to feel stronger. If they haven't already done so, people will begin to notice and ask questions.

Week 7: You will begin to see more definition on your upper abdominals.

Week 8: You will begin to see traces of definition on your front thighs.

Week 9: Your energy level jumps even higher. Your appetite for fatty foods has decreased and you begin to enjoy vegetables more.

Week 10: Your triceps will begin to feel firmer. Your waist will be smaller.

Week 11: Your body will seem to be reshaping as you look in the mirror.

Week 12: Your buttocks begin to feel tighter.

Week 13: Your stomach is getting flatter.

Week 14: Cellulite is slowly disappearing on your back thighs and buttocks.

Week 15: You make a muscle and your biceps is as hard as a rock.

Week 16: Your thighs are taking shape—harder, less flabby, more defined.

Week 17: Your stomach continues to flatten. You see more definition in your upper and side abdominals.

Week 18: You look thinner than you weigh. You can't understand it but then you remember that muscles take up less space than fat but weigh more.

Week 19: Your buttocks are clearly higher and firmer, your triceps no longer wave like a flag.

Week 20: Your entire body is shaped differently. You have clear definition on your shoulders, arms, back, and chest. Your front and back thighs are firmer and more defined. Your stomach is flatter and more defined. Your buttocks have taken a different direction—north rather than south. You are well on the way—on the lifetime road to an ever-improving body.

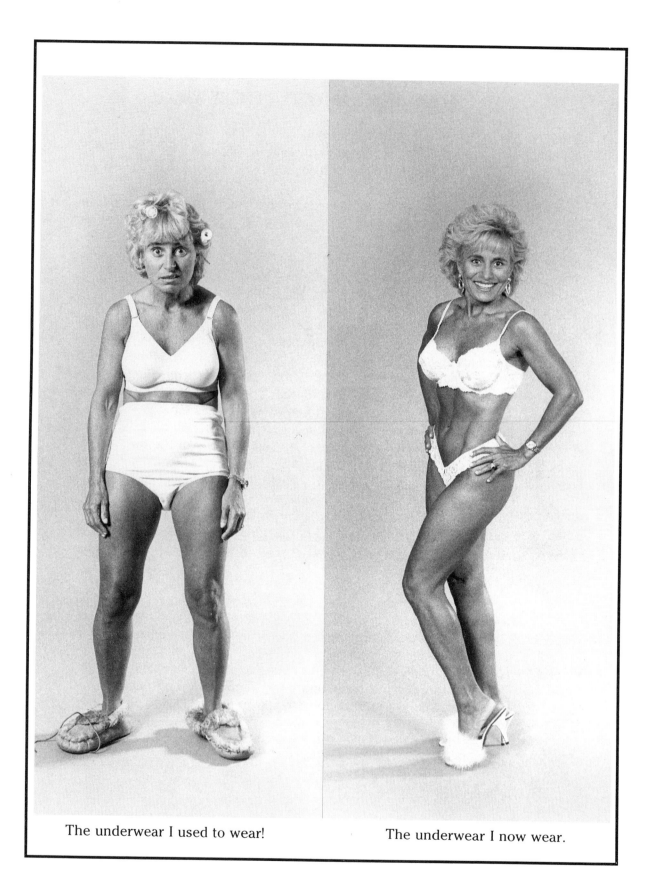

The underwear I used to wear!   The underwear I now wear.

4

"WHAT IF?"

What if I'm uncoordinated, and I don't do the repetitions exactly right?"
"What if I don't break in gently and then I can't move the next day?" "What if
I'm sore the next day even if I do break in gently?" "What if my husband wants
to join me—can a man do this workout?" "What will happen if I get sick and
stop for a while—will I have to start all over again?" "What if I'm pregnant?"

In this chapter we'll face your biggest fears and your smallest concerns and
curiosities head-on, so that no matter what situation you encounter, you'll be
ready for it: you'll be able to handle it and overcome it.

WHAT IFS—LET'S PUT YOUR MIND AT EASE BEFORE YOU START

1. What if I'm uncoordinated, and I don't do the repetitions exactly right?

Don't worry. I'm uncoordinated, and if you don't believe me, watch me perform
my demonstration the next time you see me on TV. In fact, I have a friend who
is a dancer, and after reading an early manuscript of *Definition*, and looking at
the exercise photos, and doing the workout for a week, she was doing the
movements in a more fluid and graceful manner than I. But who cares how
pretty you look? As long as you struggle along and do *your* best with the
movements, you'll see amazing progress.

2. What if I'm used to seeing things demonstrated on a video?

Be comforted by the fact that literally hundreds of thousands of women have gotten in shape by following my books with photographs and instructions alone. I have their letters and before-and-after photos (as I will soon have some of yours). But for those of you who want to see most of the exercises in this workout demonstrated, there's good news. You can get a video to show you the form, and foolish Joyce is of course the star. I move at an easy pace. After you learn the moves you will, of course, go faster. Call 1-800-433-6769 and ask for *The Bottoms Up Workout.*

3. What if I am so weak that even without weights I can only do a few repetitions of each set?

No problem. Just do those few repetitions for the first week, then increase your repetitions by two or three the next week, and keep adding each week until you are doing the full workout with no weights. Then you'll be able to do the whole workout using the one-pound dumbbells. Do that for a few weeks. Then do your first three sets with one-pound dumbbells and your last two with two-pound dumbbells for a few weeks. Finally, you'll be doing your workout using the full pyramid system of one-, two-, and three-pound dumbbells.

4. What if I don't break in gently, and I'm surprised by how out of shape I really am—and I can't move the next morning?

Don't be angry with yourself. I would say that two-thirds of my readers overestimate their ability and make this mistake—and then write to me about this problem. After reviewing the section on the difference between soreness and injury (see the following question), and checking with your doctor, unless he tells you otherwise, whatever you do, don't stop working out. You *can* move—so by an act of will, get out of bed and go on about your day (a hot shower will help). Do your workout. If you wish, you can use lighter or no weights for the next two days, and then gradually increase your weights back to where you started.

For the first five minutes of the workout, you will feel stiff and achy, but soon after that, the workout will actually be soothing and serve as a massage to your muscles. It may take a week or two, or even three, before you completely stop feeling sore. But if you stop for a week or two each time you are sore, you'll have to go through the soreness anew each time—and eventually you'll quit. So there's no way around it. Bite the bullet and get it over with once and for all. You'll live and you'll love yourself for it.

5. What if I feel sore even though I did break in gently—is something wrong with me, and how can I tell it's not an injury but just soreness?

You should feel sore even if you do break in gently—but you probably won't be so sore that you can't move the next day (as those who do not break in gently will feel). Muscle soreness is the result of microscopic tears in the fibers of the ligaments and tendons connecting the muscles, and the slight internal swelling that accompanies those tears. These tears usually occur on the stretch part of the exercise, while the muscle fibers are lengthening, yet at the same time trying to contract in order to deal with the work being required of them. These tears are not only normal but in fact necessary for muscle growth and development. Whatever you do, *don't skip working out the next day, or worse, for the next week or two* until the soreness is gone, because if you do, you will only get as sore again. It is only by working through the soreness that the muscle eventually gets strong enough to cope with the work, and the soreness disappears (unless of course, at some later date, you change your workout, go much faster than usual, or greatly and suddenly increase your weights).

If you are injured as opposed to sore, you'll know it right away. There will be an immediate warning—a sharp pain rather than a slow, gradual ache that you feel the next day. If you feel such a pain, stop immediately and see your doctor.

Common weight-training injuries are tears to the covering of the muscle (fascia injuries), tearing of ligaments, and painful inflammation of a tendon (tendinitis). If you check with your doctor before starting this workout (as you should with any new fitness regimen), and if you break in gently and use the light weights prescribed in this workout, and only gradually increase your weights, there is very little danger of injury.

6. What if I don't get sore even when I do the full workout—is something wrong with me?

I get this question once in a while and invariably I find out that the person is not doing all of the sets of all of the exercises, but rather is leaving out "unpleasant" exercises. Or the person is using too light weights (they may need three-, five-, and eight-pound weights instead of the very light one-, two-, and three-pound weights due to previous weight training and accompanying muscle strength). Or they are doing half movements—they are not reading the exercise instructions and following the photographs, but are instead making up their own version of the exercises. One final possibility is, they are moving much too slowly—which brings me to my next what if?

7. What if the workout takes me forty-five minutes when you said it should only take fifteen?

If you are doing the full split routine of two exercises per body part, five sets each, the workout should take only fifteen minutes *once you have become familiar with the movements*. The first few weeks it will naturally take longer because you have to stop and look at the photos and sometimes reread an instruction here or there, so forty-five minutes, although a bit longer than for most people, is not at all unusual.

In addition, while you are learning the movements, you will naturally move more slowly than you will once you know what you are doing. After a few weeks, your workout should speed up, and in a month (some of you much sooner, some a little longer) you should be doing the workout in fifteen minutes a day. If you're taking longer, speed up your movements. If you want to see how fast you should be going, get a copy of one of *The Fat-Burning Workout* videos (see Bibliography).

8. What if I like to do stretches before my workout—is that okay?

Yes. Although the workout provides natural warm-up sets (the first and last sets of each exercise are done with a very light weight), if you have your favorite set of stretches, and have the time to spare, by all means, stretch away.

9. What if I want to use machines instead of free weights? I happen to have a home-gym machine, and sometimes I go to a gym to work out where they have lots of machines. Is this workout as effective when done on machines—and how can I do it on a machine?

You can use machines instead of free weights for the entire workout if you wish, and, in fact, I tell you which machine to use in the exercise instructions under "Machines, etc." You can see many of the exercises demonstrated on machines in my book *Top Shape*.

It's okay to use machines for a change, but as a general rule, the free weights are superior. Not to mention convenient (free weights are cheaper: for a minimal cost you can buy them and have the convenience of working out at home)—and a simple set of free weights can take the place of twelve machines. If you do go to a gym, people will badger you if you try to monopolize two machines at a time, whereas free weights can be carried off to a corner even in a gym and hoarded.

But the greatest advantage of free weights is, they force your body to *do all of the work*, whereas a machine allows you to cheat a little. For example, machines do not allow you to go the full range of possible movement—the machine is in partial control because it stops you, depending upon the mechanism of that machine.

In a way, a machine is also like a crutch. For example, with the bench press machine, if you let go of the pressing bar, the machine will catch the weight, whereas with dumbbells, if you are doing a dumbbell press, you can't let go of the dumbbells because if you do, they will fall on you. You have no choice but to complete that repetition. In addition, knowing that a machine will catch the weight sometimes causes people to use weights they can't handle. In such a case, a person will merely jerk the weights up, and then virtually let them drop down to finish position—and as a result get very little out of the workout.

10. What if I like to go to the gym and use machines for the workout for my lower body and back—I want to put size on my thighs and widen my back—but do my upper body at home with free weights?

This is a great idea specifically in such a case, because in order to significantly widen the back (latissimus dorsi muscles), you'll need the lat-pulldown machine and the pulley row, and you might as well take advantage of the T-bar row machine. You can also do heavier bent rows by using the barbell and plates. For your legs, you will need to use the squat rack with barbells and plates and the leg-press machine. While you're at it, you might as well take advantage of the leg-extension and the leg-curl machines. (All of this is mentioned in the "Machines, etc." section of the exercise instructions.)

But if you are trying to put on size, remember that you will not be speed-supersetting. You'll have to take a rest of about thirty seconds between sets and go much heavier, and keep adding weight as you get stronger.

11. What if I've already got thinning bones—I'm sixty years old and I haven't done any weight training up until this workout. Can I reverse osteoporosis and thicken my bones with this workout?

Yes. Chances are, if you are sixty years old and you haven't done any weight-bearing exercise, you have lost bone mass. Women lose about 1 percent of bone mass a year after thirty-five, and experts are now saying that this loss doubles after menopause, so by sixty, you may have lost at least 25 percent of your bone mass, and possibly more. (Men start the loss about ten years later, and since they have thicker bones to begin with, they are not in as much danger—but yet still in some.)

But don't despair. The good news is, you can regain the bone mass you lost and, in fact, even reverse osteoporosis. Studies have been done where eighty- and ninety-year-olds who were previously unable to walk without a cane or climb stairs because of loss of bone mass were put on a weight-training program, and in a matter of months they had doubled their bone strength and were able to walk without the cane, climb stairs, and even to get up and down off the floor.

We've always known that muscles grow in response to being forced to work, but it's relatively recent news that bones grow too. But how does this happen? Bone is a living tissue composed of calcium phosphate and the protein collagen.

There are hundreds of concentric rings inside the bone (these are called haversian canals). When significant force is exerted upon a bone to which a working muscle is attached, an increased blood flow surges through the bone with nutrients. Eventually the bone builds more cells and thickens. In addition, the stress upon the bone caused by lifting weights causes an electrical charge to shoot through the haversian canals and to further stimulate the cells of the bone. In summary, it is the combination of the increased blood flow and the stimulating electrical charge that causes the bones to thicken. Don't forget what I said on page 4. My bones were tested and found to be almost twice as dense as women my age.

It must be mentioned here, however, that in addition to working out with this program, you should consume significant amounts of calcium from food, and possibly even supplement your diet with calcium pills (see page 225 for a further discussion of this).

There's one more crucial point I want to make. The beauty of this workout is, you don't just build bone in one area. Because of the nature of the workout, you are asked to stress or work nearly every significant bone in your body, so that your bones will develop in a balanced way. In other words, you won't be like a tennis player who has dense bones in her playing arm, but perhaps not anywhere else!

12. What if my husband wants to join me? Can a man do this workout? And what about teens and even children—my twelve-year-old wants to join me too.

Yes on both counts. This workout is excellent for men too—especially men who don't want bulk but just hardness and definition. However, a man who has never worked out before may be able to start with three-, five-, and eight-pound dumbbells or higher. Your husband may want to instead take advantage of the men's book I've written, *Top Shape* (see Bibliography).

If your husband or boyfriend decides to do Definition with you, let him know that he has the option of leaving out the hip/buttocks exercises (men don't have childbearing hips, and leg exercises such as squats significantly challenge the buttocks area on men).

Your twelve-year-old can do this workout too—even an eleven-year-old. If your child is younger than that most fitness experts feel it's not a good idea. In either case, you should check with your doctor first. While we're on the subject of children and teens, I must say that this workout can be a godsend for young girls who are becoming self-conscious about their figures, and in fact, it can prevent the whole bulimia/anorexia diet syndrome. I've seen hundreds of young girls who were becoming obsessed about dieting because they thought they were "fat," even though they were not, become normal happy eaters after doing this workout.

Why? As they did the workout, their bodies became harder and more well shaped and symmetrical, and they were pleased with their appearance. They no longer felt fat because, indeed, their bodies were composed of less fat and more muscle. Yes it's true. Even young girls feel fat as skinny-fats, if their bodies do not have enough muscle tone. (Your teen may prefer my youth-oriented book written with my daughter, Marthe, *The College Dorm Workout*).

13. What if my butt is already big—will this workout make it bigger than it already is?

No. The workout can only tighten, tone, and lift your buttocks because you are not using weights heavy enough to put on significant size. In order to make your butt bigger you would have to use a squat rack, a barbell, and plates, and build up to weights of over a hundred pounds.

14. What if I do this workout only one or two days a week—will it still work?

One or two days a week is better than nothing, but if you want the results I promise, you have to do it exactly the amount of time I require. If you are doing it twice a week, and doubling up for your whole body—that is to say, you are doing the thirty-minute plan, you will indeed see significant results even with working out twice a week rather than three times. However, if you are doing the fifteen-minute plan only twice a week, you won't see a whole lot of difference, but you will feel stronger and more energetic.

15. What if I get sick and have to stop for a month or two—will I lose all the ground I gained?

No. It takes as long as you worked out to outwardly lose all the ground you gained, but only one third the time to get it back. In other words, if you worked out for a year, it would take a whole year to visibly lose the muscle tone and definition you had gained, but only one third the time (four months) to regain the muscle tone and definition that you originally had. Making muscles is never a waste because the body "remembers." It's like having muscles in the body memory bank, even if you stop.

16. What if I do this workout for a year and then I decide I hate it, and I'm never going to do it again. Will all my muscles turn to fat and will I be worse off than if I never started?

No. Don't worry. Muscle cannot turn to fat. What happens is, muscle slowly shrinks back to the size it was before you started, and as discussed above, it takes about as long as you worked out for this to happen. If you eat and eat and eat, of course you will get fat, but that isn't muscle turning to fat, that is you adding fat onto your body by overeating. Of course, since your muscles will be shrinking, your metabolism will also slow down to where it used to be before you had muscle, and you'll no longer be able to eat as much as you may have become accustomed to eating.

Another point, since you won't be using up the energy you used to use working out, you'll have to find another way to spend the calories, or you'll have to further reduce your fat intake; otherwise, of course, your body will store the excess calories as fat. But none of this has to do with muscle turning to fat, and in no case will you be worse off than before. All things being equal, you will be better off, because as mentioned above, if you do decide to work out again, it will take that much less time to get in shape again.

17. What if I'm pregnant—can I still do this workout?

If you are pregnant, show this workout to your doctor and ask her how long you can continue with it. Chances are she will say that you can do it into your sixth or seventh month using the very light weights. At that time, show her a copy of my book *The 12-Minute Total-Body Workout* (see Bibliography) and ask her if you can do the workout right through your ninth month. Chances are, she will say yes.

After you have the baby, again consult with your doctor as to when you can start working out. She'll probably let you begin as early as a week to ten days after your delivery—but again, with the very light weights.

18. What if I want to get in shape for a special occasion that is coming up in only three weeks?

If you're just starting the workout, in three weeks you will absolutely start showing some clear definition, especially on your upper body—and you can show it off by wearing a shoulder-arm-back-revealing dress. In addition, you can follow the emergency Definition diet (see page 233 for this emergency diet).

19. What if I've been working out for three months and I still don't see any changes in my body?

Every six months, out of the thousands of letters I get, I'll get one like this, and invariably the person is not following the book exactly. Either she is not using any weights, or is using lighter weights, or she has not raised her weights as the workout became too easy, or she is not working out as often as she should, or she is leaving out certain exercises.

It is virtually impossible not to see significant results after three months. In any case, I implore you to take a before photo and one in three months so that at least if you write me such a letter you can show me what you are talking about. Most likely, however, you won't have that problem, and in fact, you'll be using those photos to brag to people about how much progress you have made, and if you show them to me, I may ask you to let me use them in a future book!

20. What if I want to switch around—that is to say, eat a breakfast for lunch, a lunch for dinner, and so on?

Of course you can do it. In my mind there's no such thing as "a breakfast" or "a lunch," etc. I'm concerned with your overall fat intake, that you eat often during the day, and that you get a certain amount of nutritional balance in your daily intake. You can arrange your meals as you choose.

21. What if I get bored with your meal plans—how can I improvise?

My other books have specific meal plans. As you'll see in the diet chapter, now there are no specific meal plans. Now you make up your own meals using the food lists as your guide. For delicious low-fat recipes, see the Bibliography.

22. What if I weigh myself and the scale says I didn't lose any weight—even though I look and feel tighter and more toned, and I've gone down a jeans size?

Inch for inch, muscle weighs more than fat. It takes about five inches of fat to equal the weight of one inch of muscle. Muscle is to fat as lead is to feathers. So, as your body loses fat and creates muscle, you may go down a size before you see any change on the scale. Your formerly loose, fatty body is now being condensed into tight, hard muscle that takes up less space.

If you are very overweight, of course in time you will lose weight, because you will only put a certain amount of feminine, petite muscles on your body, while at the same time you will continue to lose your excess fat. So don't worry about that cursed scale. Just do the workout and follow the low-fat eating plan, and look in the real scale—the one that is not on the floor but on the wall— the mirror.

23. What if I've been losing weight and gaining muscle tone—but then I see the scale goes up two pounds for no reason!

That's why I hate to have you weigh yourself! The body's weight fluctuates due to water retention, which fluctuates depending upon the time of the month, sodium (salt) intake, and a variety of other factors.

So what should you do—keep your sodium intake low at all times and take water pills when your period is due? No. Leave yourself alone. Keep your sodium at a normal level (see page 223), and let your body retain the water around "that time of the month." Don't fool with Mother Nature. If your body retains water when you are menstruating, it is doing it for a reason. Don't disturb the balance unless you get headaches from it, and your doctor makes a recommendation.

Water weight is not fat weight—it's very temporary. If you wanted to you could get rid of water retention naturally by cutting your sodium to a very low level for five days—and by drinking lots of water to flush out your system. (See page 233 for how to do this for a special occasion.)

24. What if I start the workout and get big muscles under my fat and I start looking even bigger than I already am—maybe I should wait until I first lose the weight?

No, no, no. A thousand times no. It is virtually impossible to get big muscles with this workout, and to in any way increase your size. Muscles take up less, not more space than fat. As you work out you will lose, not gain size as the fat goes and as you form tight, feminine, petite muscles to take the place of the bulkier fat. Believe it or not, it's true.

The worst mistake you could make would be to wait until you lose all the weight, because first of all it would take you longer to lose the weight, and losing it would feel like a punishment since you would not be working out and making muscle and feeling good about yourself. Also, once you lost the weight, you would be greatly disappointed to see that all you achieved was a flabby skinny body. So don't worry that you will get bigger, and whatever you do, don't wait until you lose the weight.

25. What if I'm on the road—do I have to carry the three sets of dumbbells?

No. You can instead either carry the one-pound weights, or no weights at all, and use the continuous tension method to replace the weights. See page 51 for a discussion on continuous tension. Another idea is to carry three-pound water weights. See page 257 to order.

26. How will my body change if I switch to this workout after having done Bottoms Up! or the Fat-Burning Workout?

If you have been doing either of these workouts, Definition will give you more overall definition, and will burn off that last bit of fat that may be lingering on your body. It will put the finishing touches on your already shapely body.

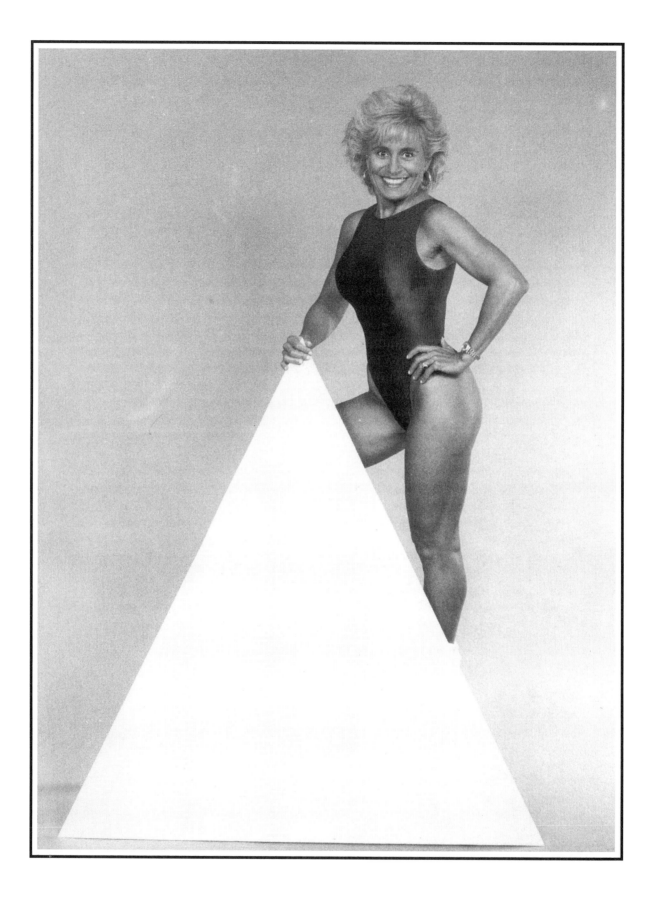

5

THE BASICS—
TERMS, TECHNIQUES, AND
EXPRESSIONS USED
IN THIS WORKOUT

In order to be able to do the workout without being held back by having to stop and say, "What does she mean by . . . ?" it's a good idea to read this chapter with a pen in your hand, underlining and making notes in the margin. This way when you encounter the terms, techniques, and expressions later on in the "How to Do the Definition Workout" chapter and "The Definition Workout" chapter itself, you won't feel threatened, but instead will feel comfortable and ready to go.

Even if you think you already know everything in this chapter, trust me, you don't. Not only do I use examples from this workout to demonstrate the terms and expressions, but I discuss new terms and expressions specifically related to this workout.

MOVING THE DUMBBELLS

An **exercise** is a specified movement for a given muscle, designed to force that muscle to become stronger and more dense, and to become reshaped. For example, the reverse curl is an exercise created to strengthen, define, and sculpt the biceps and forearm muscles.

A **repetition**, or **rep**, is one complete movement of an exercise, from start, to midpoint, to endpoint. For example, one repetition of the reverse curl involves raising one's arm with a dumbbell held palms facing the body from the down-at-the-side position to the just-below-the-shoulder position by bending the elbow (midpoint) and lowering the dumbbell back to the arm at the side position (endpoint). See page 143 for a photograph illustrating this exercise.

A **set** is a given number of repetitions of a specific exercise that are performed without a rest. In this workout, for example, you will perform fifteen repetitions of each abdominal exercise.

A **superset** is a combined set of two exercises for the same body part before a rest is taken. A **speed superset** is the same as above, only a rest is not taken until all the supersets for that body part are completed. In this workout, you will do all of your exercises in speed supersets unless you choose the option of the speed set (see below), or unless you choose to do the regular superset (a discussion of these choices is found on page 68).

For example, for your chest routine, you will speed-superset your flat flye with your flat press. You will do your first set of twelve repetitions of your flat flye, and without resting, you will do your first set of twelve repetitions of your flat press. Then again without resting you will perform your second through fifth supersets for these two exercises. A regular superset would allow the exerciser to rest a given number of seconds each time a set of the two exercises was performed. (You will also be given this option. However, if you choose it, the workout will take longer, and you lose some of the aerobic effect as well as some of your potential definition.)

The **speed set** is a combined set of all sets of one given exercise, where the exerciser only stops long enough to pick up the next weight. For example, if you are doing the Wonder Woman routine, you will speed-set rather than speed-superset the last exercise, since there is no exercise with which to superset. This will become clear as you read the individual exercise instructions in Chapter 8.

A **rest** is a pause between sets or exercises. The function of a rest is to allow the working muscle time to recover so that it can cope with the next exercise set. If your goal were to put on significant muscle mass, you would have to use relatively heavy weights, and you would need to rest about thirty to sixty seconds between each set. The purpose of this workout, however, is to burn maximum fat and deliver ultimate definition. Once you become familiar with the workout, and after you have broken in gently, and because of your use of very light weights, you will be able to breeze through your workout by taking very few rests.

WHAT YOU ARE DOING

A **routine** is the specific combination of exercises prescribed for a certain body part. For example, in this workout, the regular chest routine consists of the flat press and the flat flye. If you choose to do the Wonder Woman routine, in addition, you will be doing the incline flye. If you decide to do the Dragon Lady routine for your chest, you will also add the incline press.

A **workout** includes all the exercises to be performed by the exerciser on a given day. For example, on workout day one you will exercise your chest, triceps, shoulders, and biceps. Your workout for day two will include thighs, hip/buttocks, abdominals, back, and calves. If you choose to work out only three days a week, your workout will include all nine body parts in one day. The term "workout" can also be used to describe the overall exercise program. For example, whether you work one half of your body on workout day one, and the other half of your body on workout day two, your total workout, if you're following this program, is called the Definition workout.

The term **weight** refers to the *resistance*, or the heaviness, of the dumbbell used in a given exercise. Since this is an extreme speed workout, very light weights of one-, two-, and three-pound dumbbells (each) are recommended for beginners. The lighter weights allow you to work faster without becoming exhausted, and in addition do not require as many rests and thus keep up the aerobic, and ultra-muscle-defining, fat-burning aspects of the workout.

WHAT YOUR MUSCLES ARE DOING

A muscle is **flexed** when the muscle fibers are shortened as the muscle is squeezed together. For example, your biceps is flexed when you bend your arm. In the exercise instructions, I ask you to add to that natural flex by willfully squeezing your muscle as it flexes, adding to the force of the flex. A muscle is **stretched** when the muscle fibers are elongated or stretched. For example, your biceps muscle is stretched when you unbend your arm. In the exercise instructions, I ask you to add to that stretch by willfully letting those muscle fibers elongate to the maximum. You will be working too fast to stop and do any of this for any length of time. Flexing and stretching while working out becomes a frame of mind.

The expression **continuous tension** refers to the feeling of the weight for the fullest possible range of the movement achieved by willfully adding tension from start to finish. Maximum tension can be achieved by flexing antagonistic muscles involved in the movement. For example, when doing a biceps curl, when your arms are straight down at your sides, and your biceps are stretched to the maximum point, you begin your tension by tightening your entire arm (your triceps muscles, that work opposite or "antagonistic" to your biceps

51

muscles, will flex), and as you begin the movement, you begin the flex of the working muscle—in this case, the biceps. In other words, even though your biceps muscle is stretched, you are on the alert and the moment you begin to curl your biceps muscle, you put tension on that muscle and begin to flex it as you curl it up. Then when you reach your final curl position, you give it an extra split-second flex, called the **peak contraction**.

Since this is a speed routine, you are not going to use continuous tension and peak contraction to the extreme, in which case you would move slowly and peak-contract for a few seconds. Instead, you are going to keep up the speed of your routine, but *in the back of your mind, you will keep your eye on continuous tension and peak contraction*. However, if you are on the road and are doing the routine with no weights, you will use this method to substitute for the weights.

There are specific techniques that are an integral part of this workout. They are explained in the following paragraphs.

WHY YOU ARE BURNING FAT AND GETTING MAXIMUM DEFINITION

An **aerobic** exercise is a physical fitness activity that utilizes the larger muscles of the body, and that allows your pulse to reach a rate of 60 percent to 80 percent of its capacity, and to stay that way for twelve minutes or longer. (Some authorities insist that in order to achieve an aerobic effect one must work for twenty minutes uninterrupted; however, more and more exercise specialists are beginning to agree that one achieves an aerobic effect in twelve minutes.)

You can figure out your maximum pulse rate by subtracting your age from 220 and then multiplying the result by 80 percent. If you follow this workout exactly as prescribed, taking the minimum number of rests, you will be well within the aerobic range. You don't have to check your pulse continually. If you break into a sweat after about seven minutes, rest assured you are in the aerobic range.

An **anaerobic** activity differs from an aerobic activity in that the activity is too strenuous to be supported by the body's natural oxygen supply. When you perform an anaerobic activity such as heavy weight lifting, your body accrues an oxygen debt. When this happens you are literally forced to stop and catch your breath. Traditionally all weight training was grouped in the anaerobic category. With increasing knowledge of exercise physiology, however, fitness experts now realize that the mere appearance of a weight in a workout does not automatically classify that activity as anaerobic.

Intensity is the degree of difficulty or challenge of the exercise program you are following. Intensity can be increased by adding to the number of repetitions, increasing the load of weight, or reducing the number or length of rest periods allowed between sets and between exercises. Definition is a very high-intensity workout, because you are asked to do more repetitions by doing two extra sets for each exercise, and you are asked to work in speed supersets, which do not allow you a rest until you have completed ten sets of exercise.

Muscle isolation is the method of exercising each muscle completely and independently of other body parts. Muscle isolation is necessary in order to insure maximum muscle growth, development, and definition. In this workout you will be isolating your muscles by doing a minimum of ten sets for each muscle before moving on to the next muscle.

The **split routine** is the exercising of a given number of body parts on workout day one, and a given number of other body parts on workout day two, and so on. The purpose of the split routine is to allow the exerciser to work out two days in a row—since muscles need forty-eight hours to recuperate before being challenged again (the only exception to this rule are the abdominal muscles, this will be explained on page 96).

The **non-split routine** is the exercising of all body parts on one workout day, with the requirement that you not work with weights on the following day so that the muscles will have the required forty-eight-hour rest. (Note that one can still perform regular aerobic activities that do not require weights, either on the same day or the next day, because such activities do not tax the muscles in the same way as do weight-training exercises.)

If an exercise program has too many exercises, if the workout contains many single arm or leg movements (increasing the workout time), or if the workout requires the lifting of heavy weights, it is virtually impossible to utilize a non-split routine. The Definition workout is set up so that you can choose between the split routine or the non-split routine. See page 98 for more details. If you choose to do the Wonder Woman or Dragon Lady routines, you may find it difficult (yet not impossible) to do your entire workout in one day.

The **true (or regular) pyramid system** of weight training requires the adding of weight to each set with a simultaneous reduction of repetitions until a peak is achieved, and then the reduction of weight on each set with a simultaneous addition of repetitions until the starting amount of weight and repetitions is once again achieved. For example, in this workout, beginning exercisers will use the following pyramid:

Set 1: twelve repetitions, one-pound dumbbells
Set 2: ten repetitions, two-pound dumbbells
Set 3: eight repetitions, three-pound dumbbells
Set 4: ten repetitions, two-pound dumbbells
Set 5: twelve repetitions, one-pound dumbbells

Up until now I have always recommended the modified pyramid system which goes to the peak of the pyramid and stops. Such a system looks like this:

Set 1: twelve repetitions, one-pound dumbbells
Set 2: ten repetitions, two-pound dumbbells
Set 3: eight repetitions, three-pound dumbbells

Since I have always said that the modified pyramid system is superior to the regular pyramid system because it does not allow the muscle to become exhausted, why do I now use the regular pyramid as the mainstay of a workout system? There is really no contradiction. I have stated in other books that *fitness experts and bodybuilders use the regular pyramid system as a method of shocking the system and working harder in order to get maximum definition and to burn maximum fat, but not to build maximum muscle mass.* In other words, for our purposes in this book, maximum definition and fat burning with the development of only very moderate muscle mass, the regular or true pyramid system is ideal.

WHAT HAPPENS AS YOU GO ALONG

Progression refers to the periodic adding of weight to specific exercises when the weight being used is no longer enough of a challenge. For example, in about four weeks you may feel that you are ready to use two-, three-, and five-pound dumbbells. Two months after that, you may see that you can use three-, five-, and eight-pound dumbbells, and in another six months, you may be able to advance to five-, eight-, and ten-pound dumbbells, and so on. But where does it end? Will you eventually be lifting fifty-, seventy-five-, and 100-pound dumbbells? Of course not. This workout is too intense to allow you to do that. You will eventually reach a plateau that will be determined by your strength. I use five-, eight-, and twelve-; or five-, ten-, and fifteen-; or ten-, twelve-, and fifteen-pound dumbbells.

A **plateau** refers to a weight ceiling at which the exerciser can either remain, or attempt to break through. Most people reach their weight-training plateau in about a year. At that time you may choose to remain at that plateau or go higher. This workout is very intense, and the highest plateau most women will reach is five-, ten-, and fifteen-, or ten-, twelve-, and fifteen-pound dumbbells. If you wanted to break through that plateau, you would have to put on more size by lifting heavier weights and taking longer rests between sets for a while, and then going back to this routine with your new strength.

Training to failure means continuing a set until the muscles that are involved in that movement are so fatigued that you cannot repeat a full repetition of that movement in strict form. When you first raise your weights, you may find that the last few repetitions of your last few sets are "failure" reps. When this happens, just do the reps the best way you can, by an act of will, telling your arms or legs, or whatever body part is involved, to "Do the work!" When you train to failure, you stimulate your muscles to break a barrier and to grow and become defined. Since Definition is a very intense workout, you will often find yourself training to failure—even with the lighter weights.

THE WAY YOUR MUSCLES LOOK AND FEEL

There are certain terms that are especially important to this workout because they help you to understand exactly how your muscles will grow, develop, and become defined by this program as opposed to other workouts.

Muscle mass is the specific size of a given muscle. Moderate muscle mass growth will occur as you do the Definition workout. In order to experience muscle growth, you must consistently challenge the muscle, in isolation (that's why you are asked to do a certain number of sets for each body part before moving to the next body part), over time. Muscle mass is not only increased but shaped and sculpted by the particular work or exercise it is being asked to do.

Muscularity is a comparative term. It depicts the quantity of muscle on your body as opposed to fat. As you continue to do the Definition workout and to follow the low-fat eating plan, your muscle-to-fat ratio will increase—that is to say, you will have a higher and higher percentage of muscle, and a lower and lower percentage of fat. Your body will burn the excess fat that is under your skin and even the intramuscular fat that may have invaded your muscles over time, making them soft and less shapely.

Definition is the clearly delineated lines that separate muscles from each other and divide muscles themselves, and make them appear more shapely and attractive. Well-placed definition can also help to give the body a more balanced, symmetrical look. For example, definition in the upper back muscles draws attention away from large buttocks. Definition in the oblique (side abdominal) muscles causes the waist to appear smaller (the diagonal lines cause the waist to appear to V in and look less bulky). My waist is twenty-seven inches—that's my bone structure. No matter how thin I get, my waist will never be smaller. Yet because of my definition in that area, most people think my waist is much smaller.

When one has extreme definition, one is considered **ripped**. Right after a workout (after you have been working out for about three months), your muscles will sometimes appear to be ripped, because the blood will have been pumped into them and they will stand out to the maximum. Because of the extra blood temporarily residing in the muscle at that time, your muscles will also appear to be a little bigger than usual.

Density is the hardness of a muscle. A muscle is most dense when it has little intramuscular fat. The Definition workout will eventually force the fat not only from under your skin where most of it resides, but from the muscle itself. (Fat in a muscle can be pictured by thinking of a piece of steak that is well marbled with streaks of fat.)

Even getting rid of the fat under the skin and adding to muscle mass will cause your body to feel tighter and more toned. When you do the Definition workout and follow the low-fat diet, over time not only will you get rid of fat under the skin and add moderate muscle mass, you will eventually remove the fat marbling from the muscle itself, and that increasing muscle density will make your muscles feel even more firm to the touch.

Total body **symmetry** refers to the balance and proportion of all the muscles on your body in relation to all the other muscles on your body. The Definition workout will improve your body symmetry in that it will build moderate muscle mass where needed and give ideal definition to your overall musculature.

Some women insist upon only exercising their stomach, buttocks, hips, and thighs. They will not have total body symmetry, since their upper body will appear out of balance. Such women will have flabby triceps (the part of the arm that appears to wave like a flag once a woman passes forty), sloping shoulders to begin with, as I did, because of genetics (see my photograph on page eleven of *Bottoms Up!*) or as muscle atrophies over the years, and so on, while their lower bodies will appear tight and toned and well shaped. In addition, a shapely, well-developed lower body will make an out-of-shape upper body look even more emaciated and out of shape. For this reason, it is not a great idea to pick and choose which body parts to exercise. It is, however, okay to do special work to bring a lagging body part up to par. A discussion of this is found on page 96.

EQUIPMENT NEEDED FOR THIS WORKOUT

The only equipment you will need for this workout is three sets of dumbbells and a bench or step. You will be doing the exercises at home with free weights (dumbbells are considered free weights because they can be freely carried about, as opposed to machines that are stationary and bound to the floor).

If you want to use a home-gym machine, or if you want to do the workout in a gym using machines, you will have that option. However, if you work out in a gym you will probably have to use speed sets rather than speed supersets unless the gym is rather empty (otherwise you may find it difficult to keep vigilance on the two machines at a time that you will need to monopolize for this workout).

A **dumbbell** is a short bar (usually made of metal, but sometimes made of plastic and filled with sand—not my favorite kind) that can be held in one hand and that has a permanently fixed ball-shaped raised section on each end. Dumbbells also come in take-apart sets, where you can add weights to each end. I do not recommend them because it takes too much time to change the weights. In the case of this workout, you would not have the time, and in fact, it would seriously slow you down and significantly defeat the efficacy of the workout.

You will need three sets of very light dumbbells for this workout: ones, twos, and threes. Note that whenever I say "a set of . . ." I mean each dumbbell. For example, a set of one-pound dumbbells means two dumbbells of one pound each. A set of two-pound dumbbells means two dumbbells of two pounds each. A set of three-pound dumbbells means two dumbbells of three pounds each. This definition was universally accepted until recently when certain merchants decided to emphasize the total weight in order to make the customer see how much she was getting for her money (a set of two-pound dumbbells weighs four pounds, for example).

For your convenience, I can send you the sets of one-, two-, and three-pound dumbbells, neatly packaged and all prepaid, shipping included, and later, heavier dumbbells, or you can get them in any gym equipment store (where they will be the least expensive), or in a sporting goods store (see page 257 for more information).

The **flat exercise bench** is a long, narrow, padded bench that is parallel to the floor, and is built specially for exercise. The flat bench can be made to go to an incline by placing two telephone directories (tape them together so they won't slip) under one end of the bench.

The flat/incline/decline exercise bench is the same as a flat exercise bench, only it can be raised to a 45 degree angle so that you can do certain exercises (in the case of this workout, the incline flye and incline press if you are doing Wonder Woman or Dragon Lady routines). It also has a foothold so that you can do decline presses or flyes, or decline sit-ups or crunches.

Substitutes for a bench. A bench is always safest because it is made specifically for many of the exercises described in this workout. However, if you simply cannot get a bench at this time, you may be able to use a piano bench or a cocktail table (assuming the edges are flat). Another option is a step such as the one used in step aerobics. (See exercise photos on pages 117 and 119 for example.)

WHY BOTHER WITH THE DESCRIPTIONS OF THE MUSCLES INVOLVED IN THIS WORKOUT?

While you are doing the workout, I want you to think about the specific muscle you are exercising and to consciously "work with" that muscle, "telling" it to get stronger, firmer, more shapely, and more defined. In order to do this, you will have to get a picture of where the muscle is, and it would help if you knew how that muscle worked and exactly where it is located on your body. Later, when you read the exercise descriptions, it is also very important that you think before you start the workout, "I am exercising my _____ muscles." For example, before I knew what I was doing, I remember how I used to go to a health spa and use the bench press machine. As I was pressing away, since you use your arms to push the bar up and down, I assumed I was working my arms. In the meantime, everyone (except me at the time) knows that the bench press is a chest exercise.

"So what if you didn't know what you were exercising," you might argue. "Is it really a big deal?" Yes. I was thinking that my arms should do the work, so I was consciously pushing the bar up with my arm muscles, whereas if I had realized that my chest muscles should be doing the work, I would have made a conscious effort to let my pectoral (chest) muscles take as much of the responsibility for the work as possible. In fact, you will improve your workout by 100 percent if you realize which muscles are doing the work, and if you make it your business to let that muscle do the work by visualizing it working and by willfully flexing and stretching that muscle as it goes through the start, midpoint, and finish aspects of the movement.

The following descriptions of the muscles are described in the order that they are found in the workout.

Chest
(Pectoralis Major—Pectorals, or "Pecs")

The pectoralis major is a two-headed, fan-shaped muscle that lies across the front of the upper chest. It originates at the collarbone and runs along the breastbone to the cartilage connecting the upper ribs to the breastbone. The clavicular head, which is the smallest of the two heads, forms the upper pectoral area, while the larger sternal head forms the lower pectoral area. The pectoral muscles in women are covered by fatty tissue (breasts). To increase breast size, one must actually gain fat in this area (and most women do go up a bra size when they put on significant weight). However, breast size can appear to increase if one develops the pectoral muscles—since they are located under the breasts. In addition, well-developed chest muscles give the chest muscles definition, which creates more cleavage.

The pectoralis muscles function to flex the chest and to pull the upper arm down and across the body.

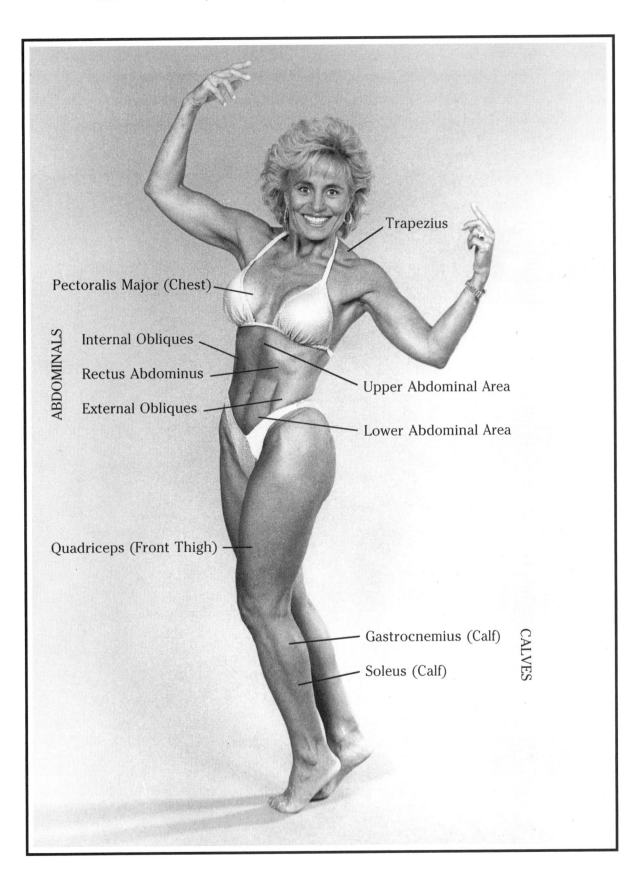

Trapezius

Pectoralis Major (Chest)

ABDOMINALS

Internal Obliques

Rectus Abdominus

External Obliques

Upper Abdominal Area

Lower Abdominal Area

Quadriceps (Front Thigh)

Gastrocnemius (Calf)

CALVES

Soleus (Calf)

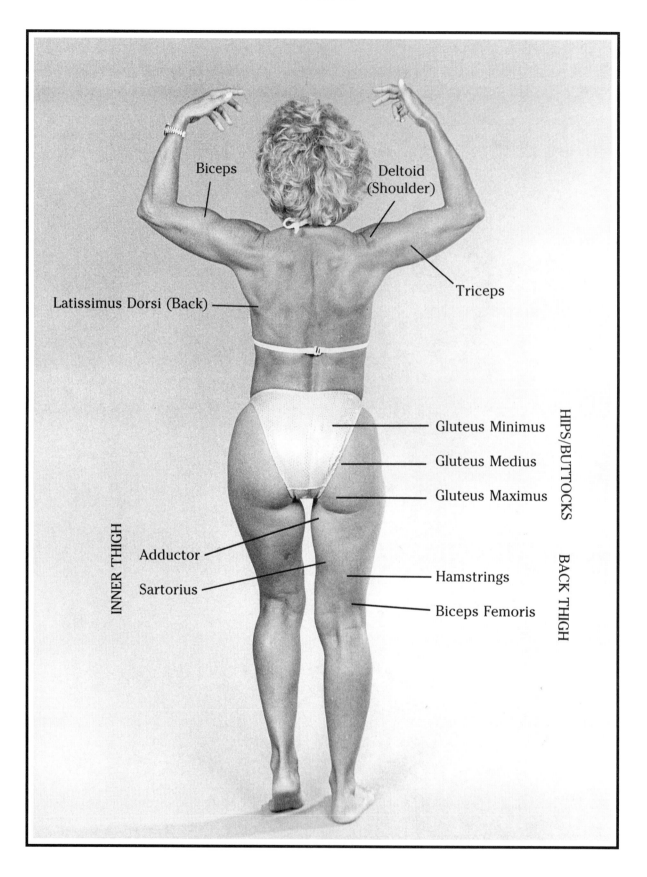

Biceps

Deltoid
(Shoulder)

Triceps

Latissimus Dorsi (Back)

Gluteus Minimus

Gluteus Medius

Gluteus Maximus

HIPS/BUTTOCKS

BACK THIGH

INNER THIGH

Adductor

Sartorius

Hamstrings

Biceps Femoris

Triceps

The triceps is a three-headed muscle (hence the name "triceps"). This muscle is the notorious "flag waver" when flabby and out of shape. (It usually begins to happen as a woman ages unless she does something to rebuild the muscle.) The triceps is located on the underside of the arm, just opposite the biceps muscle.

One of the three heads of this muscle attaches to the shoulder blade, while the other two heads originate from the back side of the upper arm and insert at the elbow. The longer head functions to pull the arm back once it has been moved away from the body, while the other two heads, in conjunction with the longer head, work to extend the arm and the forearm.

Shoulder
(Deltoid)

The deltoid is a triangular muscle that looks like an inverted delta, the Greek letter (hence the name "deltoid"). It consists of three parts, which can function independently or as a group: the anterior (front) deltoid, the medial (middle or side) deltoid, and the posterior (rear) deltoid.

The entire deltoid muscle originates in the upper area of the shoulder blade, where it joins the collarbone. The three parts of the muscle weave together and are attached on the bone of the upper arm. One angle drapes over the shoulder area, another points down the arm, weaving around the front of that arm, and the third drapes down the back of the arm.

The anterior deltoid cooperates with the pectoral muscles to lift the arm and to move it forward. The medial deltoid helps to lift the arm sideways; and the posterior deltoid works in conjunction with the latissimus dorsi to extend the arm backward.

Biceps

The biceps is a two-headed muscle (hence the name "biceps") with one short head and one long head. Both heads originate on the cavity of the shoulder blade where the upper arm bone inserts into the shoulder. The two heads join to form a "hump" about a third of the way down the arm. The other end of the biceps is attached to the bones of the forearm by one connecting tendon.

The biceps works to twist the hand and to flex the arm.

Front, Inner, and Back Thigh
(Quadriceps, Sartorius, Adductor, and Biceps Femoris, or Hamstrings)

The quadriceps, or front thigh muscle, consists of four muscles (hence the name "quadriceps") that run along the thigh and end at the kneecap. The four muscles are the rectus femoris, which originates on the front of the hipbone, and the vasti (three muscles grouped together: the vastus lateralis, the vastus medialis, and the vastus intermedius), which originate on the thighbone.

The entire quadriceps group works to extend the leg.

The sartorius runs along the inner thigh, from the hipbone to the inside of the knee. It is the longest muscle in the human body. It functions to rotate the thigh.

The adductor muscles are also located on the inner thigh. This muscle group originates from the lower pelvic area on the pubis bone and rises to the shaft of the thighbone, where it is inserted. This muscle group works in cooperation with other inner thigh muscles to flex, rotate, and pull the legs together from a wide stance.

The hamstring (biceps femoris) muscle group is located on the back thigh. It consists of two muscle groups—the semimembranosus and the semitendinosus. They originate in the bony area of the pelvis and end along the back of the knee joint. This muscle group works to bend the knee.

Hips/Buttocks
(Gluteus Maximus, Gluteus Medius, and Gluteus Minimus)

The largest of the gluteus muscles, the gluteus maximus, originates from the iliac crest of the thighbone and runs down to the tailbone. It works to extend and rotate the thigh when extreme force is needed, as in climbing the stairs.

The gluteus medius is located just beneath the gluteus maximus. It functions to raise the leg out to the side and to balance the hips as weight is transferred from one foot to the other.

The gluteus minimus originates on the iliac crest of the hipbone and performs the same function as the gluteus medius.

Many women ask me, "What about exercises for the outer thigh?" The hips include the outer thigh, and all hips/buttocks exercises also shape and tone the outer thigh.

Abdominals
(Rectus Abdominus, External Obliques, and Internal Obliques)

The rectus abdominus is a powerful long muscle that is segmented (hence, when developed, the "beer can," or ripped, appearance). The abdominal muscles originate from the fifth through seventh ribs, and run vertically across the abdominal wall. They work to pull the upper body toward the lower body when sitting up from a prone position.

Technically speaking, the rectus abdominus is one long muscle, but because it is necessary to isolate the upper from the lower areas for workout concentration, most people speak of "upper abdominals" and "lower abdominals."

The external oblique muscles originate at the side of the lower ribs and run diagonally to the rectus abdominus. The obliques are attached to the sheath of fibrous tissue that surrounds the rectus abdominus. The obliques work with other muscles to rotate and flex the torso.

The internal oblique muscles run at right angles to the external obliques and beneath them. It is this angle that forms the angle of the waistline, and determines how big or small your waist is (all other things being equal—that is to say, assuming that you are not overweight with excess fat in the way).

Back
(Latissimus Dorsi and Trapezius)

The latissimus dorsi originates along the spinal column in the middle of the back and runs upward and sideways to the shoulders, inserting in the front of the upper arm. These muscles work to pull the shoulder back and downward and the arm toward the body.

The most visible of the back muscles, well-developed latissimus dorsi muscles help to give the back a V-shaped look, which in turn helps to give the hips and waist a smaller look.

The trapezius is a triangular muscle that originates along the spine and runs from the back of the neck to the middle of the back. The upper fibers of the trapezius are attached to the collarbone and show visible outward development in the neck-shoulder area, but this showing is only, in a manner of speaking, the tip of the iceberg, because in reality the hidden part of the trapezius muscles descend all the way down to the lower spine.

Calf
(Gastrocnemius and Soleus)

The gastrocnemius is a two-headed muscle that connects the middle of the lower leg and ties in with the Achilles tendon. The juncture where the two muscles tie together forms what is visibly the calf.

The gastrocnemius muscle works in opposition to the extensor muscles of the lower leg, which pull the foot upward. It also works with other muscles to bend the knee and flex the foot downward.

The soleus muscle originates on the back of the tibia and head of the fibula bones. It lies just beneath the gastrocnemius muscle, but does not pass the knee joint, so that it functions only to flex the foot downward, but cannot help to bend the knee.

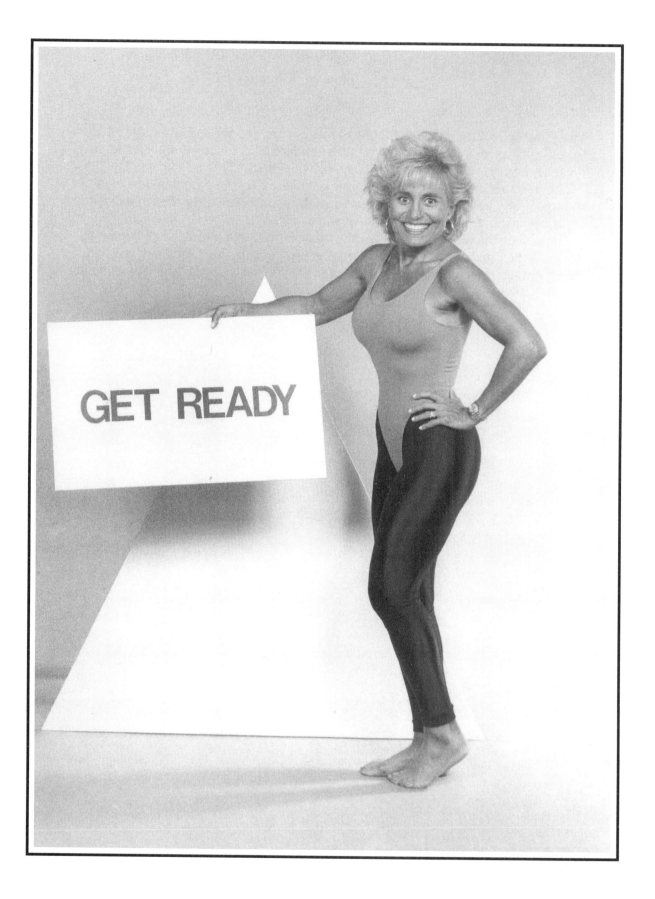

GET READY

6

HOW TO DO THE DEFINITION WORKOUT

Definition is a powerful workout. You work quickly, taking almost no rests at all, and in this sense it is the most aerobic of all my workouts—and the fastest moving. You virtually have no time to think about it—once you pick up that first weight, it's one, two, three, four, five supersets—a fifteen-second rest, and on to the next exercise. Before you know what hit you, you're finished. You can't believe it happened so quickly—and *it will* happen quickly once you have broken in gently.

In this chapter you'll learn how to perform the Definition workout. You'll find out how much work to do if you are on the fifteen-minute, six-day-a-week plan, or how much work to do if you are on the thirty-minute, three-day-a-week plan, and you'll learn how to add in the Wonder Woman and Dragon Lady exercises if you want extra work for an even greater challenge.

THE REGULAR DEFINITION WORKOUT: FIFTEEN MINUTES SIX TIMES A WEEK, OR THIRTY MINUTES THREE TIMES A WEEK

The regular workout has only two exercises per body part—only two are needed because you do five sets of each exercise—ten sets in all. This adds up to one set more than you would have done had you used any modest bodybuilding routine, where you do three exercises, and three sets each for each body part—a total of nine sets.

You have a choice as far as how many days a week you want to work out. You can either break the workout up into halves, doing it in fifteen-minute segments six days a week, or you can exercise your entire body on each workout day, in which case the workout will take you thirty minutes. But the bonus will be you will only have to work out three days a week!

The Basis of This Workout: The True Pyramid System and the Speed Superset

This workout is based upon the true pyramid system and the superset. If you've used a regular bodybuilding program, you realize that the typical way to work out is to perform about three exercises for a body part, and to perform about three sets of each of those exercises. In this type of routine, you would do all three sets of one exercise before moving to the next exercise, and you would rest thirty to sixty seconds between each set.

When performing the Definition workout, however, you will be using the true pyramid system—and you will also use the superset. But since you will take no rests until you have completed five supersets, you will be doing the speed superset. In other words, you will do two things different from the typical bodybuilding routine: 1) instead of doing only three sets per body part, you will do five sets per body part. 2) instead of completing all five sets for one exercise before advancing to the next exercise for that body part, you will continually switch back and forth from your first exercise for that body part to your second exercise for that body part, without resting, until you have completed all five supersets, ten sets in all. At this point, you will have completed your entire routine for that body part, and will be allowed to rest for only fifteen seconds before advancing to the next body part.

Let's take a look at how this works for the chest routine.

CHEST ROUTINE

1. Flat flye
2. Flat press

TRUE PYRAMID SYSTEM

Set 1: twelve repetitions, one-pound dumbbells
Set 2: ten repetitions, two-pound dumbbells
Set 3: eight repetitions, three-pound dumbbells
Set 4: ten repetitions, two-pound dumbbells
Set 5: twelve repetitions, one-pound dumbbells

You do your first set of twelve repetitions of the flat flye with one-pound dumbbells; then, while still lying on the bench (or step), you do your first set of twelve repetitions of the flat press with the same one-pound dumbbells. Without resting, you drop the one-pound dumbbells and pick up the two-pound dumbbells, and do your second set of ten repetitions of the flat flye, and again, while still lying on the bench (or step), and without resting, you do your second set of ten repetitions of the flat press with the same two-pound dumbbells.

Without resting, you drop the two-pound dumbbells and pick up the three-pound dumbbells and do your third set of eight repetitions of the flat flye, and again, while still lying on the bench (or step), and without resting, you do your third set of eight repetitions of the flat press with the same three-pound dumbbells. (Now you are ready for the big challenge—you are about to descend the pyramid without resting, so . . .)

Without resting, you drop the three-pound dumbbells and pick up the two-pound dumbbells and do your fourth set of ten repetitions of the flat flye, and again, while still lying on the bench (or step), and without resting, you do your fourth set of ten repetitions of the flat press with the same two-pound dumbbells. (Now you are approaching your final set.)

Without resting, you drop the two-pound dumbbells and pick up the one-pound dumbbells, and do your fifth set of twelve repetitions of the flat flye, and again, while still lying on the bench (or step), and without resting, you do your fifth set of twelve repetitions of the flat press. Now you rest fifteen seconds and begin the next body part.

You will work in the same manner for all body parts that require weights: chest, triceps, shoulders, biceps, thighs, back, and calves. Let's take a closer look.

General Application for Workout Day One: Chest, Triceps, Shoulders, Biceps, Thighs, Back, and Calves

Set 1: Twelve repetitions for each of two exercises—no rest between sets. Use one-pound dumbbells.

No rest before beginning set 2.

Set 2: Ten repetitions for each of two exercises—no rest between sets. Use two-pound dumbbells.

No rest before beginning set 3.

Set 3: Eight repetitions for each of two exercises—no rest between sets. Use three-pound dumbbells.

No rest before beginning set 4.

Set 4: Ten repetitions for each of two exercises—no rest between sets. Use two-pound dumbbells.

No rest before beginning set 5.

Set 5: Twelve repetitions for each of two exercises—no rest between sets. Use one-pound dumbbells.

Rest fifteen seconds and then begin your next body part!

After you have completed your **chest** routine, the first body part of workout day one, you will rest fifteen seconds and move to your next body part, your **triceps**. You will speed-superset the entire routine in the same manner, going back and forth between your first triceps exercise, the seated overhead press, and the second triceps exercise, the close bench press, until you have completed all five supersets (ten sets in all) without having rested once.

Then you will rest fifteen seconds and move to your next body part, your **shoulders**, working in the same manner and speed-supersetting your first shoulder exercise, the reverse overhead lateral, with your second shoulder exercise, the bent lateral, until you have completed that routine.

You will then rest fifteen seconds and move to your last body part of the day (if you are on the fifteen-minute workout), your **biceps**, speed-supersetting your first biceps exercise, the simultaneous standing curl, with the second biceps exercise, the alternate reverse curl.

Don't Panic

Don't throw this book across the room thinking, "This is crazy. I can't understand it." A picture is worth a thousand words, and I have laid out the workout in exactly the form you will be doing it (see Chapter 8). I also remind you of sets, reps, and weights for each exercise. But do read this chapter anyway. Later, the combination of the words you read here and the photographs and reminders you see in Chapter 8 will take you right through the workout.

WORKOUT DAY TWO FOR THE FIFTEEN-MINUTE, SIX-DAY-A-WEEK WORKOUT (TO BE CONTINUED ON WORKOUT DAY ONE FOR THE THIRTY-MINUTE, THREE-DAY-A-WEEK WORKOUT)

You will continue to work in the same manner as above, speed-supersetting your first exercise for the **thighs**, the squat (or the substitute if you have bad knees), with your second exercise for the thighs, the leg extension, until you have completed all five speed supersets.

Supersetting Body Parts That Require No Weights

Now you come to your **hips/buttocks** routine, where no weights are used. Speed supersetting remains the same. You continue to switch back and forth between the first and second exercises. But what about the pyramid system? Well, since there are no weights involved, we can't very well pyramid them, so instead we will maintain a steady fifteen repetitions for each exercise. Here's how it will look.

You do your first set of fifteen repetitions of the prone floor scissors, and without resting, you do your first set of fifteen repetitions of the second hips/ buttocks exercise, the prone butt lift.

Without resting, you go back to your first exercise for that body part, the prone floor scissors and again do fifteen repetitions, and again, without resting, do fifteen repetitions of the second exercise for your hips/buttocks area, the prone butt lift. You do three more speed supersets as above, for a total of five speed supersets.

Now you do your **abdominals**. Once again, no weight is involved, so you will work in the same manner as you did with your hips/buttocks routine—doing fifteen repetitions for each set, and switching back and forth from the first and second exercises in the routine until you have completed all five speed supersets, ten sets in all.

Your next body part is your **back**, and since you use weights, you will of course return to the same system you used for chest, triceps, shoulders, biceps, and thighs.

Finally, you do your **calves**. Since you use weights, you will continue with the same system you used for your chest, triceps, shoulders, biceps, thighs, and back.

Review of Exercises and Their Order in the Regular Definition Workout

1. Chest	6. Hips/Buttocks
Flat flye	Prone floor scissors
Flat press	Prone butt lift

2. Triceps	7. Abdominals
Seated overhead press	Alternate knee-in
Close bench press	Knee-raised crunch

3. Shoulders	8. Back
Reverse overhead lateral	Double-arm bent row
Bent lateral	Seated back lateral

4. Biceps	9. Calves
Simultaneous standing curl	Seated straight-toe calf raise
Alternate reverse curl	Seated angled-out-toe calf raise

5. Thighs
Squat (or side leg lift)
Leg extension

If you are doing the fifteen-minute, six-day-a-week plan, exercise body parts one to four on workout day one, and exercise body parts five to nine on workout day two. Repeat the sequence two more times for a total of six workout days in a week. If you are doing the thirty-minute, three-day-a-week plan, exercise body parts one to nine on workout day one. Rest a day and repeat the sequence two more days, leaving a day of rest between, for a total of three workout days in a week.

THE WONDER WOMAN WORKOUT: TWENTY-TWO-MINUTE SIX-DAY-A-WEEK PLAN, OR FORTY-FOUR-MINUTE THREE-DAY-A-WEEK PLAN

The Wonder Woman Definition workout is exactly the same as the regular Definition workout, except you do a little more work by adding one exercise to each body part. However, since there will now be an "odd fellow" in each body part, there will be no "partner" with which to superset this new man in town. So you will simply speed-set the third exercise.

The Speed Set

The speed set is very simple. You take no rests between the sets of a given exercise, but instead speed right along to the next set in that exercise. Since there are five sets for each exercise of this workout, it means that you will be doing all five sets of the exercise before taking a fifteen-second rest.

Let's see how this works. Here is the Wonder Woman chest routine.

WONDER WOMAN CHEST ROUTINE

> Flat flye
> Flat press
> Incline flye

You will perform all five of your flat flye and flat press exercise speed supersets going back and forth between your flat flye and your flat press until you have completed those two exercises. Then you will take a fifteen-second rest and speed-set your lone incline flye, doing all five sets of your incline flye without resting. Of course you will use the full pyramid system as described on page 68.

But what about body parts that don't use weights? Nothing changes. You will work as above, speed-supersetting your first two exercises by switching back and forth until you have completed all five supersets, and then take a fifteen-second rest and move to the lone speed set. Let's look at a body part that does not require the use of weights, the hips/buttocks routine.

WONDER WOMAN HIPS/BUTTOCKS ROUTINE

Prone floor scissors
Prone butt lift
Horizontal scissors

You will speed-superset your prone floor scissors by doing fifteen repetitions of that exercise and then, without resting, doing fifteen repetitions of the prone butt lift, and repeating that sequence four more times until all five supersets have been performed. Then you will rest fifteen seconds and speed-set your lone horizontal scissors. You will perform five sets of fifteen repetitions each of the horizontal scissors without resting. (In other words you will do seventy-five repetitions, fifteen times five, of the horizontal scissors without resting. Yes, it's murder. But you won't die and the fat will burn!)

The Wonder Woman Definition Workout

Here is a list of all the exercises in the Wonder Woman Definition workout. You will note that the first two exercises are the same as the regular workout, and that one exercise has been added for each body part.

1. Chest

Flat flye
Flat press
Incline flye

2. Triceps

Seated overhead press
Close bench press
Simultaneous kickback

3. Shoulders

Reverse overhead lateral
Bent lateral
Side lateral

4. Biceps

Simultaneous standing curl
Alternate reverse curl
Lying simultaneous flat-bench curl

5. Thighs

Squat (or side leg lift)
Leg extension
Leg curl

6. Hips/Buttocks

Prone floor scissors
Prone butt lift
Horizontal scissors

7. Abdominals

Alternate knee-in
Knee-raised crunch
Alternate twisting knee-in

8. Back

Double-arm bent row
Seated back lateral
Upright row

9. Calves

Seated straight-toe calf raise
Seated angled-out-toe calf raise
Standing straight-toe calf raise

If you are doing the twenty-two-minute, six-day-a-week plan, exercise body parts one to four on workout day one and exercise body parts five to nine on workout day two. Repeat the sequence two more times for a total of six workout days in a week. If you are doing the forty-four-minute, three-day-a-week plan, exercise body parts one to nine on workout day one. Rest a day and repeat the sequence two more days, leaving a day of rest between, for a total of three workout days in a week.

THE DRAGON LADY WORKOUT: TWENTY-NINE-MINUTE SIX-DAY-A-WEEK PLAN, OR FIFTY-EIGHT-MINUTE THREE-DAY-A-WEEK PLAN

The Dragon Lady Definition workout is exactly the same as the regular Definition workout, only you do double the work of that workout. Instead of doing only two exercises per body part, you do four exercises per body part. This makes for a very neat combination of exercises, because you can speed-superset your first two exercises for each body part as you did in the regular workout, and in the same manner speed-superset your second two exercises for each body part. Let's take a look at the chest routine to see how it works.

THE DRAGON LADY CHEST ROUTINE

Flat flye
Flat press
Incline flye
Incline press

You will perform all five of your flat flye and flat press speed supersets together without resting. Then you will take a fifteen-second rest and you will perform all five of your incline flye and incline press speed supersets. Then you will take a fifteen-second rest and move to the next body part, the triceps routine.

You will work in the same manner for all nine body parts, speed-supersetting your first two exercises, taking a fifteen-second rest, speed-supersetting your next two exercises, and taking a fifteen-second rest, and moving to the next body part, and so on.

Here is a list of all of the exercises in the Dragon Lady workout. You will notice that they include all the exercises of the regular and Wonder Woman workouts, with one exercise added to each body part.

If you are doing the twenty-nine-minute, six-day-a-week plan, exercise body parts one to four on workout day one, and exercise body parts five to nine on workout day two. Repeat the sequence two more times for a total of six workout days in a week. If you are doing the fifty-eight-minute, three-day-a-week plan, exercise body parts one to nine on workout day one. Rest a day and repeat the sequence two more days, leaving a day of rest between, for a total of three workout days in a week.

The Definition Dragon Lady Workout

1. Chest

Flat flye
Flat press
Incline flye
Incline press

2. Triceps

Seated overhead press
Close bench press
Simultaneous kickback
Lying extension

3. Shoulders

Reverse overhead lateral
Bent lateral
Side lateral
Alternate shoulder press

4. Biceps

Simultaneous standing curl
Alternate reverse curl
Lying simultaneous flat-bench curl
Lying alternate flat-bench hammer curl

5. Thighs

Squat (or side leg lift)
Leg extension
Leg curl
Frog-leg front squat

6. Hips/Buttocks

Prone floor scissors
Prone butt lift
Horizontal scissors
Standing butt squeeze

7. Abdominals

Alternate knee-in
Knee-raised crunch
Alternate twisting knee-in
Side leg raise

8. Back

Double-arm bent row
Seated back lateral
Upright row
Double-arm reverse row

9. Calves

Seated straight-toe calf raise
Seated angled-out-toe calf raise
Standing straight-toe calf raise
Standing angled-in-toe calf raise

WHY SUCH LIGHT WEIGHTS—AND WHEN TO RAISE YOUR WEIGHTS

Due to the intensity of the workout, most people should start out with the very light dumbbells of one, two, and three pounds. However, those of you who have been using much higher weights for one of my other workouts may go a little higher. For example, if you have advanced to five, ten, and fifteen in either the Fat-Burning Workout or Bottoms Up! you can use three, five, and eight pounds to begin with.

A good rule of thumb is to cut your weights down to half of what you used to use, and then very, very gradually build up as you get stronger. But don't think for one moment that cutting your weight means that you are getting less out of the workout. The lower weights are more than compensated for by the intensity of the workout—you are going soooo much faster. As mentioned before, this is the most intense and aerobic of all my workouts.

In time, when the weights you are using become too inconsequential a challenge, and you seem to get little or no resistance from them, and they are in fact nearly flying through the air, it is time to raise your weights—but very gradually. Let's see how this looks.

Beginning Weights

Set 1: one-pound dumbbells
Set 2: two-pound dumbbells
Set 3: three-pound dumbbells
Set 4: two-pound dumbbells
Set 5: one-pound dumbbells

Raising Weights the First Time

Set 1: two-pound dumbbells
Set 2: three-pound dumbbells
Set 3: five-pound dumbbells
Set 4: three-pound dumbbells
Set 5: two-pound dumbbells

Raising Weights the Second Time

Set 1: three-pound dumbbells
Set 2: five-pound dumbbells
Set 3: eight-pound dumbbells
Set 4: five-pound dumbbells
Set 5: three-pound dumbbells

Raising Weights the Third Time

Set 1: five-pound dumbbells
Set 2: eight-pound dumbbells
Set 3: ten-pound dumbbells
Set 4: eight-pound dumbbells
Set 5: five-pound dumbbells

Raising Weights the Fourth Time	Raising Weights the Fifth Time
Set 1: eight-pound dumbbells	**Set 1:** ten-pound dumbbells
Set 2: ten-pound dumbbells	**Set 2:** twelve-pound dumbbells
Set 3: twelve-pound dumbbells	**Set 3:** fifteen-pound dumbbells
Set 4: ten-pound dumbbells	**Set 4:** twelve-pound dumbbells
Set 5: eight-pound dumbbells	**Set 5:** ten-pound dumbbells

Notice that the weight raising is very slow, and never overall. You always simply eliminate the first and lightest weight, and instead begin with what used to be your set two weight. Take a look at the above examples and you'll see what I mean. For example, the first time you raise your weights, you eliminate the one-pound dumbbells for set one, and instead start out with the two-pound dumbbells. You do your second set with the three-pound dumbbells, and when you come to your third set, you need to use a higher set of dumbbells, in this case five pounds (for some reason, they don't make four-pound dumbbells).

But what about other weight combinations? For example, can there be a five-pound gap between the weights? The answer is yes only if you are already a seasoned weight trainer and switching to this program. For example, if you worked yourself up to ten, fifteen, and twenty pounds in the Fat-Burning Workout or Bottoms Up! you may not feel like buying more than one set of dumbbells, so instead of cutting your weight in half and using five, eight, and ten, which would require you to purchase both five- and eight-pound dumbbells, you may decide to use five, ten, and fifteen pounds for this workout right away.

But whatever you do, don't push it. If in doubt, it's better to invest in the extra set of dumbbells (they are not very expensive when you compare them to the price of machines or gym memberships). In short, it is much better to start out a little too light and work your way up than to start out a little too heavy and then become discouraged and find yourself saying, "Is Joyce crazy? This workout is impossible." I would hate to see this happen, especially when the fact is, if you started out with very light weights, you could do this with no problem and love it—and in fact, I would like to see everyone do the workout with the one-, two-, and three-pound dumbbells for the first week or two at least, no matter how well trained they are in weight training and aerobics. (I'm a realist, however, so in good conscience, I give you all of your options.)

How Often Will You Raise Your Weights?

Everyone is different, but a good rule of thumb is, you should begin to ask yourself if you can raise your weights after three to six weeks. Then you may stay at the same weights for two or three months, or more. The next time you raise your weights may be in two to six months. The point is, be alert to the need to raise the weights. Be sensitive to the feeling that the weights are as light as feathers and seem to fly through the air with little resistance. You don't want that to happen. You want to feel as if you are working.

The Highest You Should Go

Unless you are a professional bodybuilder, the highest you should go is the fifth weight raising in the table above: ten, twelve, and fifteen—and frankly, I doubt if any of you will want to go that high. A much more realistic goal is the fourth weight raise, eight, ten, and twelve (or five, ten, and fifteen if you have opted not to purchase the extra set of dumbbells). In any case, you would probably not reach your highest weight for at least a year.

Buttocks and Abdominals Require No Weights

As mentioned before in this chapter, the hips/buttocks and abdominal exercises require no weights. These two areas are famous for fat accumulation—and need more repetitions in place of using weights. For this reason, instead of using weights and the true pyramid system, you will simply do fifteen repetitions of each exercise, and you will superset back and forth, bouncing from your first and second exercises for that body part.

Those of you who are familiar with my other workout books may wonder why I am now not offering you the option of doing fifteen to twenty-five repetitions per exercise for the hips/buttocks and abdominals. The answer is simple. Because of the intensity of the workout, it is not realistic to ask you to go higher than fifteen repetitions per exercise. Frankly, there would be no harm done if you could manage to go up to twenty-five repetitions per exercise, but I tried it, and felt overworked. But if you do it and love it, please write to me and tell me about it.

If You Only Have One Set of Dumbbells and Want to Start Now

This workout is so exciting when you do it with the three sets of dumbbells of one, two, and three pounds because you never get bored; your body is coaxed into going from one set to the other because it knows that it will get some sort of a change with each set. However, suppose you already have a set of three-pound dumbbells at home, and you don't feel like buying anything more, and want to use that set for all five sets of each exercise?

You can do that, but you'll run into three annoyances: 1) Both your mind and body will be bored by the tedium of using only one weight, so you'll have to use real discipline to go on. 2) You will be more exhausted because you'll be using the heavier three-pound weight for all three sets. 3) You will be in danger of forgetting how many sets you did, since there will be no automatic marker of the set by the heaviness of the weight.

I suggest that you order the set of one-, two-, and three-pound dumbbells but begin the workout with what you have while you're waiting. (The sets I offer are prepacked and cannot be separated, so if you already have three-pound dumbbells, I can't just send you the one- and two-pounders. I have extra three-pound dumbbells around, and I end up lending them to friends who want to start a workout. So if you end up with extra threes, they will probably come in handy someday.)

BREAKING IN GENTLY

Your break-in plan will depend upon what you've been doing up until this point. Obviously, if you're not in aerobic shape, and, you've never worked out with weights before, you will have to take it a little slower than someone who is in such shape. If you're somewhere in between, you'll have to take a midway course. The following paragraphs will guide you along.

Breaking In if You Have Already Been Working with Weights and Are in Aerobic Shape

If you have been recently following the workout described in either of my books *The Fat-Burning Workout* or *Bottoms Up!* you are ready to do this workout with no break-in period if and only if you either use the one-, two-, and three-pound dumbbells or at least cut your previous weight load in half. Why must you reduce your weight so drastically?

This is a much more intense workout than either of the above, and as you will quickly see, much more exhausting if you try to do it with the same weights you used before. It is, as mentioned before, the most aerobic of all my workouts.

If you are in aerobic shape (you run, bike, swim, or some such thing), and you have been following a regular weight-training workout such as is found in *Now or Never* or *The 12-Minute Total-Body Workout*, you may or may not be able to just jump into this workout, even if you either use the one-, two-, and three-pound dumbbells or cut your weights in half, because you have not yet combined aerobics with weight training. Try it, but if you find that you're exhausted, take fifteen-second rests between each superset, rather than performing all five supersets of a given body part before resting. Each time you work out, try to eliminate one of the extra fifteen-second rests, until you are working as prescribed in the beginning of this chapter (resting fifteen seconds only after a body part has been completed).

Breaking In if You Have Already Been Working with Weights but Are Not in Aerobic Shape

If you've been following a regular workout with weights, but are not in aerobic shape, you can do the workout using one-, two-, and three-pound dumbbells or slightly higher, but you'll have to rest fifteen seconds between each superset for the first week. The next week, you can feel it out and try to rest only one extra time per body part. For example, you may perform two supersets, rest fifteen seconds, and perform the other three supersets, and then take your legitimate fifteen-second rest before moving to the next body part. By the third week, you should be able to perform the entire workout as described in the instructions at the beginning of this chapter.

I must give you fair warning here. If you try to use weights such as five, ten, and fifteen or heavier, you will have to take many more rests than allowed. Even if you are used to working with ten-, fifteen-, and twenty-pound dumbbells, it is much better to use the very light dumbbells and work your way up to the higher weights (which will happen very quickly in your case, since you are strong due to previous training).

You will be thrilled with the results of this workout because your already formed muscles will start to show fantastic definition in a matter of weeks.

Breaking In if You Are in Aerobic Shape, Are Basically Strong, but Have Little or No Experience in Working with Weights

When you add in the weights, be sure to use the one-, two-, and three-pound dumbbells.

Week 1: Do the entire workout with no weights, following the true pyramid system exactly as if you were using weights. For example, you will still do twelve repetitions for your first superset of two exercises, ten repetitions for your second superset of two exercises, eight repetitions for your third superset of two exercises, ten repetitions for your fourth superset of two exercises, and twelve repetitions for your last superset of two exercises. Then you will take a fifteen-second rest and move to the next body part. You will do this until you complete the workout.

Week 2: Do set one of each exercise. (You will be supersetting your first two exercises, and doing twelve repetitions of each exercise with the one-pound dumbbells.)

Week 3: Do sets one to three of each exercise. (You will be supersetting your first two exercises, and doing twelve repetitions for your first superset with the one-pound dumbbells, ten repetitions of your second superset with the two-pound dumbbells, and eight repetitions of your third superset with the three-pound dumbbells.

Week 4: You are on the full program. Do all five supersets for each body part as described in the beginning of this chapter.

Breaking In if You Have Never Worked with Weights, Are Not in Aerobic Shape, and Are Very Weak

Actually, this is the perfect workout for you, because it will get you into both aerobic and strength shape quickly—and it's not overwhelming because you are using such light weights. You'll progress more quickly than you could ever have imagined. When you add in the weights, be sure to use the one-, two-, and three-pound dumbbells.

Week 1: Do set one of each exercise, with no weights. (You will be supersetting your first two exercises, and doing twelve repetitions of each exercise with no weights.)

Week 2: Do sets one to three of each exercise with no weights. (You will be supersetting your first two exercises, and doing twelve repetitions for your first superset, ten repetitions of your second superset, and eight repetitions of your third superset.)

Week 3: Do the entire workout, all five supersets of each exercise, with no weights.

Week 4: Do one set of each exercise using the one-pound weights. You will be supersetting your first two exercises and doing twelve repetitions of each exercise with the one-pound dumbbells.

Week 5: Do two sets for each exercise using the one- and two-pound weights. You will be supersetting your first two exercises and doing twelve repetitions of each exercise for your first set with the one-pound dumbbells, and without resting, your second set of ten repetitions of each exercise with the two-pound dumbbells.

Week 6: Do the first three supersets for each exercise, using the one-pound weights for the first superset, the two-pound weights for the second superset, and the three-pound weights for the third superset. You will be supersetting your first two exercises and doing twelve repetitions of each exercise for your first set with the one-pound dumbbells, and without resting, your second set of ten repetitions of each exercise with the two-pound dumbbells, and without resting, your third set of eight repetitions of each exercise with the three-pound dumbbells.

Week 7: You are on the full program. Do all five supersets for all exercises. Work exactly as described in the beginning of this chapter.

WHAT IF YOU CAN'T GET THE MINIMUM NUMBER OF REPETITIONS FOR A GIVEN SET?

If you find yourself unable to do the minimum number of repetitions for any given set, start out with as much as you can handle—say, three repetitions per set; just do what you can and try to add one repetition each week. For example, when doing the abdominal workout, chances are you will only be able to do three to five repetitions per set in the beginning. This is fine. Just do what you can, and each week, try to add one repetition per set until you come up to the full number of repetitions for each set.

WHAT IF YOU NEED TO TAKE MORE RESTS THAN ARE ALLOWED?

After the break-in-gently period, you are allowed a rest only after you have speed-supersetted two exercises using the full pyramid system. In other words, you will have done ten sets without resting—quite a tall order.

If you feel that you need more rests, you may take them. Here's how. Take a rest after each superset—say, a five-to-fifteen-second rest. Then you will have simply supersetted, rather than speed-supersetted your workout. This will lengthen your workout by five to ten minutes, but no harm will be done. You will also lose slightly some of the aerobic effect.

USING THIS WORKOUT TO PUT ON MORE SIZE

This is not the ideal workout to use to add muscle size, but you can use it to add moderate size if you take the rests as described above, and increase your weights as you get stronger—using three, five, and eight; five, eight, and ten; ten, twelve, and fifteen (-pound dumbbells) and so on. A better way to put on more size is to read Chapter 10 and switch to one of those workouts.

MACHINES, ETC.

You will note that in the exercise instructions I tell you which machines and other equipment can be used in place of a given exercise. For those of you who want to use these substitutes, fine. The only problem you may have is, most machines have only ten-pound weight gradations, so you will probably have to keep your weight at the lowest for all five supersets until you become strong enough to raise the weights as prescribed. Then, the highest you will probably go is ten, twenty, and thirty pounds.

GIVE IT TIME—THE WORKOUT TAKES LONGER IN THE LEARNING STAGES!

I get so many letters from women who say, "It took me nearly double the time you said it would take to do the workout. What's wrong with me?" In the past, I foolishly assumed that everyone would realize that, of course, in the beginning stages, in the learning stages, the workout will take you a little longer, because you are still looking at the photographs and trying to make sure you're doing the workout correctly. After a few months, the workout will be as promised, only fifteen minutes, or in fact, sometimes shorter. And this time I've included a tear-out chart so you can see an overview of all the exercises (see pages 191–201).

MOVE IT!

But this brings me to my next, and most important point—one that I have also neglected to emphasize in any other book. Of course if you're going to work like a snail, it's going to take you twice as long to do the workout—and in the bargain, you won't burn as much fat. After you know what you're doing, please, by all means, move it! None of this prolonged, tedious, slow-motion action—but rather rapid-pace, deliberate, quick-fire repetitions—and yes, without cutting the movements short. It can be done.

STRETCHING

Before starting your workout, if you wish, you may do a few repetitions of each exercise for the entire routine without weights. But since your first set will be very light—you will be using a one-pound dumbbell—you will probably feel, as I do, that the stretch is included in the first set, and that taking the time to do additional stretches in the case of this workout is unnecessary.

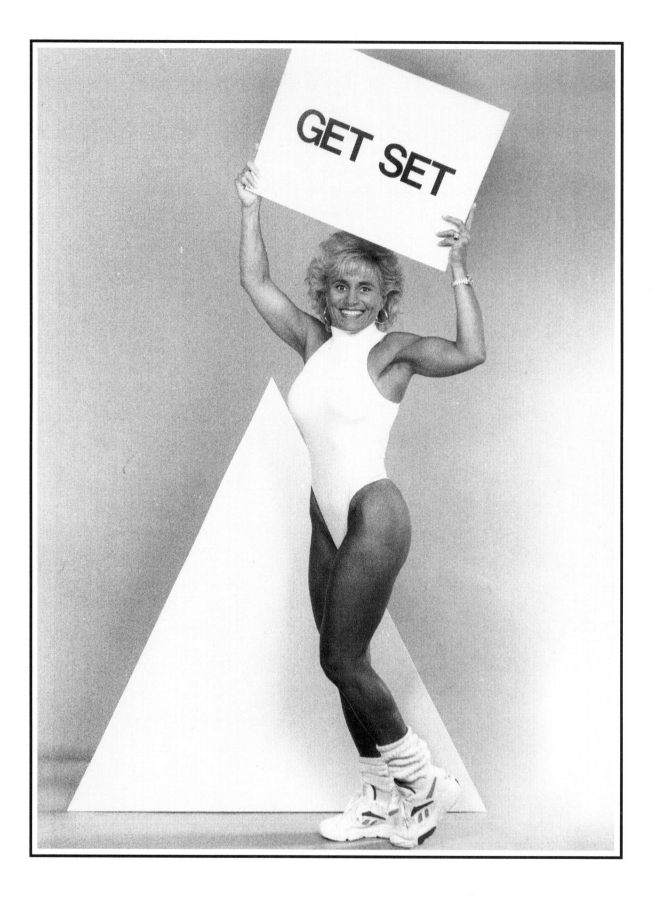

7

WORKOUT PLANS, EXTRA AEROBICS, AND MOTIVATION

You know just about everything you need to know. You're ready to start. But perhaps before you do, it would be a good idea to think of your options as far as workout plans go. What if you want to do the fifteen-minute plan and nothing else? What if you want to do the fifteen-minute plan but still continue with a favorite aerobic activity? Suppose you want to do the thirty-minute plan and no extra aerobics—or the thirty-minute plan with extra aerobics? You could probably figure it out for yourself, but in case you need a little help, this chapter will spell it out for you. Finally, before you actually start the workout found in the next chapter, I'll provide some motivation to get you started and to keep you going when the going gets tough.

First we'll talk about how the Definition workout is in and of itself an aerobic activity, and then we'll discuss additional aerobic options, so that you can decide which, if any, additional aerobic activities you want to add to your weekly workout plan.

WHAT IS AN AEROBIC ACTIVITY, AND WHY IS THE DEFINITION WORKOUT ALMOST PURE AEROBICS?

Until recently, most experts believed that in order to be considered aerobic, an exercise regimen must involve the movement of the large muscles of the body in a continuous rhythmic motion *for twenty minutes or more*, and that the activity must keep the pulse rate up between *60 percent and 80 percent of maximum capacity* for the duration of that time. In the past few years, however, fitness experts are coming to agree that an activity is aerobic if the activity continues for *twelve minutes* or more, and the pulse rate is kept up to *60 percent or higher of maximum capacity*.

The Definition workout keeps your pulse rate up to 60 percent or higher of capacity, and requires you to work for fifteen minutes or more (depending upon which plan you have chosen). The only reason one might raise a question as to the aerobic nature of the Definition workout is the fifteen-second rest taken four times during the fifteen-minute workout, or nine times during the thirty-minute workout. It is these meager rests that cause me to say "almost" pure aerobics, because as mentioned above, technically speaking, there should be no rests at all. However, the extreme intensity of the workout more than compensates for the very short rests, and in fact anyone who has done this workout tells me that it is more challenging than any aerobic workout they have ever done!

ADDING AEROBICS TO YOUR WORKOUT FOR ADDITIONAL FAT BURNING AND HEART–LUNG STRENGTHENING

If you only have time to do one thing—aerobics or the Definition workout—the Definition workout wins hands down, because it tightens, tones, shapes, strengthens, and defines your body while at the same time it burns fat and strengthens your heart and lungs. In short, if you chose to do an aerobic activity to the exclusion of the Definition workout, you would be making a *BIG mistake.* Why?

An aerobic activity's main power is to strengthen the heart and lungs, and to burn fat. Only as a side effect does it shape a body part or two—depending upon the specific nature of that activity. For example, if you run, you will have shapely calves. That's it. If you stair-step, you'll have a strong hip/butt/thigh area, but not even shapely thighs (you have to work with weights to sculpt those muscles). If you jump around in a general aerobics class you'll lose some overall body fat, but you will reshape nothing! And so it goes. You name it—I'll call it. No matter which aerobic activity you do, you will never ever, not in a million years be able to reshape your body, or for that matter, to get the feminine, pretty definition that makes you look so sexy. The only way you can reshape your body is by working with weights in a scientific fashion the way bodybuilders do—but with lighter weights and for less time (as described in any of my workout books, for example).

So why do extra aerobics at all? Why not just throw them out the window? No. If you have the time, and if you want to burn additional fat, and further strengthen your heart and lungs, extra aerobics are wonderful. In fact, since I love to eat, I try to incorporate extra aerobics into my weekly plan, but if I'm pressed for time, and it comes down to one or the other, for the reasons discussed above, I will *always* put my weight workout first.

MONITORING YOURSELF TO SEE IF YOU ARE IN THE AEROBIC RANGE

If you know me at all, by now you know that I think monitoring is an unnecessary distraction. However, if you want to monitor your pulse rate out of curiosity, or because you want to make sure that you're in the ideal fat-burning range of 60 percent to 70 percent of capacity, here's how to do it.

You must determine your minimum, medium, and maximum aerobic pulse rate. In order to do this, subtract your age from 220, then multiply the result by 60 percent. This will give you the minimum ideal rate for your fat-burning aerobic range. Now multiply the figure by 70 percent. This will give you your medium pulse rate, but the maximum ideal range for fat burning. If you multiply the number by 80 percent, this will give you your maximum pulse rate—the highest safe aerobic range—and in my opinion, higher than is ideal for fat burning. The research keeps changing, but most experts agree that we burn the most fat when we are between 60 percent and 70 percent of our maximum range.

If you're not going to monitor yourself, how will you know if you are in the ideal fat-burning range? It's simple. After about five to seven minutes, you should break a sweat. You should not be so out of breath that you can't answer a question, but you should find it a little uncomfortable to carry on a conversation.

AEROBIC EXERCISE CHART

Aerobic Activity	Calories Burned in 15 Minutes
Definition workout	210
Stair machine	195
Running eight-minute mile	172
Swimming	157
Rope jumping	150
Low-impact aerobics	150
NordicTrack	125
Trampoline jumping	125
Race walking	120
Cross-country skiing	115
Rowing machine	110
Stationary bike riding	110
Walking at fast pace	80

It is important to note that your actual fat-burning rate will depend upon how vigorously you perform the exercise. The above chart assumes that you are working at a vigorous pace.

BREAKING IN GENTLY WITH AN AEROBIC ACTIVITY

If you are not in aerobic shape (that is, you are not already doing some aerobic activity for approximately fifteen minutes or more), you should break in gently using the following guidelines:

Week 1: three to five minutes
Week 2: five to seven minutes
Week 3: seven to ten minutes
Week 4: ten to fifteen minutes
Week 5: fifteen to twenty minutes
Week 6: twenty to twenty-five minutes
Week 7: twenty-five to thirty minutes

(Continue to work in this manner if you wish to build up to longer aerobic periods.)

Work from the lower end of each week's range upward, so that by the end of the week you have achieved the highest number of minutes. For example, on the first day of week one, you may bike for three minutes. The next day you bike for four minutes, and so on, until by the end of the week you are riding for five minutes. The next week you begin at five minutes and gradually work your way up to seven minutes by the end of the week, and so on.

CHOOSING YOUR EXTRA AEROBIC ACTIVITY

When it comes to deciding which aerobic activity you will choose, there are only two rules of thumb: do what you like and what your physical condition will allow. For example, if you hate the water, why torture yourself by forcing yourself to swim—unless of course, due to physical limitations, it is the only aerobic activity your condition will allow, and you are determined to burn extra fat.

I enjoy riding the exercise bike and at the same time keeping up with what's happening on the talk shows. It doesn't matter if I'm home when they are on. Since I know that I will be riding my bike for about thirty minutes, I systematically tape shows for that purpose.

I also love walking, now that I have a British bulldog. (They say dogs and their owners begin to look alike—you should see him, he's all muscle. You can see him if you are curious, as he's featured with my daughter in her book, *The College Dorm Workout.*) Instead of riding the bike, I'll drag the poor cur along for about fifty minutes (that's about his limit).

Another aerobic activity I like is jumping rope. It makes me feel like Rocky training for his big fight. I jump rope when it is really the only convenient aerobic activity I can do—for example, when I'm on the road for weeks at a time and often in hotels that have no aerobic facilities, or if I just don't feel like making contact with the human world until after I've had my morning coffee. I can do it in my room while watching the morning news.

I used to run, and I loved it, but I must confess running finally caught up with me. I began to get driving pains at night in my hips, knees, and ankles. I experimented by stopping the thirty-minute runs, and sure enough, the pains stopped. But thank God, there are a host of other aerobic activities I can do if I choose to do the extra aerobics.

Ideally, when it comes to aerobics, it's a good idea to vary your activity rather than do the same thing each day. Do I vary my aerobic activity? I never used to do that but I'm trying now. I'll walk one day, ride the stationary bike the next, and use the stair-stepper the next, and occasionally I'll jump rope. By varying the activity you reduce the risk of abusing any one specific joint area, and at the same time you prevent your body from becoming so used to the exercise that you lose some of its effect.

WORKOUT SCHEDULES—FROM MINIMUM TO MAXIMUM

There's only one way to make sure that you get your workouts in and that's to plan them into your weekly schedule. In order to do this, you'll have to get yourself a wall calendar or a desktop weekly planner and write them in exactly when you plan to do them.

The Definition Minimum Plan with No Extra Aerobics

There are two workout options, the fifteen-minute, six-day-a-week plan, or the thirty-minute, three-day-a-week plan; here they are:

THE FIFTEEN-MINUTE WORKOUT

Sunday	Monday	Tuesday	Wednesday	Thursday	Friday	Saturday
Rest	Upper	Lower	Upper	Lower	Upper	Lower

THE THIRTY-MINUTE WORKOUT

Sunday	Monday	Tuesday	Wednesday	Thursday	Friday	Saturday
Rest	Total Body	Rest	Total Body	Rest	Total Body	Rest

The Definition Middle-of-the-Road Plan with Moderate Extra Aerobics

THE FIFTEEN-MINUTE WORKOUT

Sunday	Monday	Tuesday	Wednesday	Thursday	Friday	Saturday
Aerobics	Upper	Lower Aerobics	Upper	Lower Aerobics	Upper	Lower

94

THE THIRTY-MINUTE WORKOUT

Sunday	Monday	Tuesday	Wednesday	Thursday	Friday	Saturday
Rest	Total Body	Aerobics	Total Body	Aerobics	Total Body	Aerobics

(See how neat this thirty-minute plan is. If you love aerobics, you can have the best of both worlds.)

The Definition Maximum Plan with Maximum Extra Aerobics

THE FIFTEEN-MINUTE WORKOUT

Sunday	Monday	Tuesday	Wednesday	Thursday	Friday	Saturday
Aerobics	Upper	Lower Aerobics	Upper Aerobics	Lower Aerobics	Upper Aerobics	Lower Aerobics

(Note that it's a good idea to take one day off a week from aerobics in order to prevent injury, but it doesn't matter that you do aerobics on the same day that you do the Definition workout.)

THE THIRTY-MINUTE WORKOUT

Sunday	Monday	Tuesday	Wednesday	Thursday	Friday	Saturday
Aerobics	Total Body Aerobics	Aerobics	Total Body Aerobics	Aerobics	Total Body	Aerobics

(Reminder: Take a minimum one day off a week from aerobics.)

Doing Extra Work for Your Stomach

Many people want to do extra work for the abdominal area, and as you know, you can in fact exercise that body part almost every day. In this workout, the abdominals are included in the lower body workout. But what if you want to work your abdominals more often? First, try increasing the quantity of your abdominal exercises by adding in both Wonder Woman and Dragon Lady exercises for this body part. If you still feel that you need extra work, I want you to get a copy of *Gut Busters* (see Bibliography) and do the seven exercises in that book on the days you don't do abdominals for this workout, for a total of a six-day-a-week abdominal workout. (Even your abdominals deserve one day off a week.) Another alternative is to do the *Bottoms Up Workout: Middle Body* video (see Bibliography) on the alternate days—or even every day—replacing the Definition stomach workout completely.

Doing Extra Work for Your Hips/Buttocks/Thigh Area

Many women need extra work for the hips/buttocks/thigh area, but you cannot exercise these body parts two days in a row because like all muscles except abdominals, they need forty-eight hours to recover from a weight workout for ideal development.

If you need extra work for this area, first try adding in both Wonder Woman and Dragon Lady exercises for these body parts. If you still feel that you need more work, then do my Bottoms Up! workout for hips/butt/thighs, replacing that workout for hips/butt and thighs in this workout, but do all of your other body parts using this book. Since there are seven exercises for each of these body parts in *Bottoms Up!* you will add about ten minutes to your workout time (see Bibliography).

Making Up Your Own Workout Schedule: Basic Rules of Thumb

You can alter the above schedules in any way you want, except you must observe the following rules:

1. Never work the *total body* two days in a row.
2. Never work the *upper body* two days in a row.
3. Never work the *lower body* two days in a row.

What can you do two to six days in a row if you please?

1. Any aerobic activity (even on days you worked upper body, lower body, or both).
2. Abdominals.

What if You Are Doing the Wonder Woman or Dragon Lady Routines?

Easy. You simply follow any of the plans above—only, of course, your workout time will be longer. How much longer will depend upon whether you do Wonder Woman, which adds about seven minutes to your fifteen-minute routine, bringing it up to twenty-two minutes, and fourteen minutes to your thirty-minute routine, bringing it up to forty-four minutes.

If you are doing the Dragon Lady routine, you will add about fourteen minutes to your fifteen-minute routine, bringing it up to about twenty-nine minutes, and twenty-eight minutes to your thirty-minute routine, bringing it up to about fifty-eight minutes. (It is difficult to predict your exact times—and remember, the times assume you are used to the workout and are working at full speed. This will happen in about three to four weeks after you have broken in gently—but then you'll have it for life, so be patient.)

Which Plan Is Better: The Fifteen-Minute, Six-Day-a-Week Plan, or the Thirty-Minute, Three-Day-a-Week Plan?

Which plan you choose will often depend on your schedule. You may need those four free days for other business, or you may just like to get it over with more quickly, or you may want to free up those other four days for aerobics.

On the other hand, you may be the type of person who has to do something every day (like going to work from Monday through Friday) in order to establish and keep a habit. Breaking the regimen up into Monday, Wednesday, and Friday may be bad for you, because having that day off in between may make you not want to go back to work (back to the workout) the next day.

Everyone is different. Think about yourself and try the plan that seems most suited to you. Once you are working out for a while, there's no reason why you can't switch back and forth whenever you feel like it—from the fifteen-minute to the thirty-minute plan and vice versa.

Making Up a Missed Workout

If you miss a workout, you can make it up, but you'll have to remember the above rules about making up a workout: you can't exercise the upper or lower body two days in a row. This means for example, if you are on the fifteen-minute plan, and you miss the upper body, and the next day you are scheduled to do the lower body, you can of course do both. But when the following day comes along, and the upper body is due, you can't do it because you exercised the upper body the previous day. You'll have to take a day off and work the whole body the next day.

Your best bet, if you are on the fifteen-minute plan, is to simply let it go and do the body part that is due for that day (if you skipped a few days, do the body part that you did not do last, but it won't really matter a whole lot if you can't remember which it was).

If you are on the thirty-minute plan and you skip a workout, you can work your total body the next day. For example, if you usually work your total body on Mondays, Wednesdays, and Fridays, but miss your workout on Monday, you can do it on Tuesday instead. But on Wednesday, when your total body workout is again normally due, you'll have to rest or do an aerobic activity, and wait until Thursday to do your workout. Then on Friday, when your total body workout is again due, you'll have to take off or do an aerobic activity and do your total body workout on Saturday. You'll again have to take off Sunday or do an aerobic activity. On Monday you will be back on schedule!

MOTIVATION

Before you get to the next chapter, the actual workout, I think we should talk about motivation, so that we can head off any problems that you may have in either getting started or following through with your plans.

You've got great intentions. You were very excited when you first heard about this workout. You bought the book, and you read it from cover to cover. You even underlined things and made notes in the margins, the way I asked you to do. You've even marked your calendar for the whole month to schedule in your workouts. But it's one thing to read about something, and to plan something, and quite another to do it—as scheduled, day after day, without giving in to the temptation to be lazy, to get discouraged, and to eventually just plain quit. What can you do when thoughts assail you, thoughts that would ordinarily stop you from working out on a given day, or even stop you from working out forever?

I know how it feels to be discouraged and to be tempted not to work out. I had to go through all of the mental battles before I went on "automatic," and even now, from time to time I have to fight myself, but the battle is much much easier now—more like when you feel like calling in sick to work. You think about it, but then you say, "No. I'd better just drag myself there. Once I'm on my way I'll be happy I didn't give in," and you go. Here are some tips, some "shots in the arm," for you if you are tempted to not get started in the first place, are enticed to skip a workout, or are tempted to quit permanently.

What to Do if You Just Can't Get Started in the First Place

When you first picked up this book, you were motivated. Even though you had already tried and failed at so many diets and shape-up plans, this one sounded different and you thought, "Why not?" But now that it's time to start, you're getting cold feet. You're thinking, "I can't put myself though another failure." Or you're thinking, "Hmm. If it only takes fifteen minutes a day—how could it work? It was wishful thinking. I'm not going to waste my time!"

Or you may be dreading the break-in period. "I'll have to think about what I'm doing every minute," you imagine. "At least with my old workout I was on automatic—I didn't have to think about anything." Or worse: "I haven't exercised in years. This may kill me." And finally, you may attack yourself with thoughts such as, "How do I know I'll stick to this—I'm such a quitter."

First of all, don't blame yourself for feeling this way. Most people go through a cold-feet period just before starting something new—especially if the new endeavor is very important to them, or if they have failed in that area before. For example, you should have seen me when I first decided to take up ballroom dancing!

Believe it or not, I've always thought of myself as uncoordinated, and in addition, dense when it comes to learning dance steps. I'm sure it relates back to kindergarten, when for the life of them, neither my mother nor my teacher could get it though my thick skull that skipping is different from galloping. No matter what they did, I would trot like an uncoordinated pony—all the while trying with every brain cell I could muster to force my feet to do the skipping motion. Eventually I learned to skip, but it left me with a permanent lack of confidence when it came to anything that required physical coordination.

But I had always admired ballroom dancing—you know, the Fred Astaire and Ginger Rogers kind of dancing. I particularly had in mind the waltz, the peabody (a very fancy dance done in the 1940s to Andrews Sisters–type music), and the tango.

I made an appointment with a renowned dance studio and was excited at the prospect of learning to dance. All week I bragged to my friends, "I'm taking up ballroom dancing." But the day I was supposed to go I started thinking about what a klutz I was, and canceled my appointment. The next day I felt badly about it and realized that I still really wanted to learn to dance, and I made another appointment. Again I was tempted to cancel, but by an act of will I forced myself to go. The dance lesson was quite pleasant, but as expected, I was a slow learner. The next lesson time came, and I had to fight myself not to call and cancel. I dreaded appearing stupid and feared I would look the fool when I couldn't remember one single thing from the last lesson. But I did show up and the teacher patiently reviewed. Slowly I began to learn and to retain what I had learned. But I still had to fight my temptation to cancel at least every other lesson. Finally, in time, I began to look forward to dance lessons. Not only did I learn to dance, but I learned to overcome my fear of it. I did a demonstration waltz and peabody in front of my entire dance school, and although I still don't have perfect posture, my feet were steppin' and I looked pretty good, if I do say so myself.

The point is, it's normal, as I've said, to pull back just before starting something new—especially if you've failed at it before, and if you seriously doubt that you can do it, and even more so if you want it so bad you can almost taste it, because your strong desire magnifies the disappointment you imagine you will feel if you do fail. It's normal to think these thoughts, but you can get past them. Just acknowledge the thought, and go ahead and do what you planned to do anyway.

It may be the seeming enormousness of the project that is turning you off. I get letters from women all the time who tell me that the mere thought of looking at the pictures and learning all the new moves was enough to give them a headache. They tentatively forged ahead, at first feeling zero confidence that they were doing the exercise movements correctly. These women end their letters by asking if I would be interested in bringing them on a television show so that they could strut their before-and-after selves.

Not for Any Price—They'd Rather Fight Than Quit

There's no pressure on you. No one is monitoring you. You can take your time, do this at your own pace. Who cares if it takes a while to get it. You can't put a price on it once you have it. In fact I've asked women who have done this for a year and gone from fat and flabby to femininely muscular and sexy how much I would have to pay them if we could magically take away the workout and put them back in their former shape, but with the condition that they could never do this, or any other workout like it, again. "No way, not for any price," they say. "Not for all the tea in China," they cry. "I would rather fight than switch," they proclaim. And they're not kidding. And you and I know why. To get this body thing conquered once and for all is worth more than money. It's worth your peace of mind, your self-esteem, and your energy—your very life.

Don't worry that you failed at other diets and workouts. Many of them were failure-bound because they asked you to starve, or they gave you foolish exercises that could never reshape your body—that did not give you a systematic way to put sexy muscle in all the right places. Or you might not have been psychologically ready to get in shape. Or the workout may have been asking you to devote too much of your time to it. This is a new day. Anything can happen.

The big key is to open the book, and start to do the movements. In fact, you can do one repetition of each exercise in the entire workout just to get an overview of what you'll be doing. This will help calm you down and make you feel more in control.

I don't care how many other things you've quit. This time you're going to make it. In fact, at least 90 percent of my letters come from women who failed at every other workout and diet, and succeeded with one of mine. But the only way to get the process in the works is to get started, so open up to Chapter 8, and calmly start doing one repetition of each exercise. Then open up to page 81, break in gently, and decide which break-in plan you will use, and begin your workout for the day. A few minutes into the workout you'll wonder why you were so hesitant.

What to Do if You've Been Working Out a Few Weeks and Are Thinking of Quitting Because You're Not Seeing the Results You Had Dreamed of.

Look at Chapter 3. Read the stories of the before-and-after women. Some of them were thinking of quitting for the first month or two because they didn't see the results they thought they should see. But they didn't. They plodded on, and look at them now.

Everyone is different. You can read the guidelines in Chapter 3, "What You Will See and Feel Week by Week," and find your category, but the fact is, each individual is so unique that her body will develop at its own pace. Most likely, you'll be most impatient with your stomach, your hips/buttocks area, and your thighs. These often take much longer to kick in, but once they do, it's for ever.

You may even have an unusual problem. Whereas most women's upper body develops quickly—arms, upper back, shoulders, chest—your arms may take longer to show results than most people's. You may say to yourself, "What's wrong with me? I must be the exception. I'm the one person for whom this workout won't work." But just keep going. Eventually *it will* work on you—and in time every single part of your body will come up to par.

You can't go by the immediate. If you've been doing the workout exactly as described in the book, and a year from now you tell me you don't see results, write to me and I'll talk with you on the phone at my own expense and see why. But this has never happened. Why? Because any woman who has done the workout for that long has seen even greater results than she could have imagined. Believe me, you will not be the exception, but you must hang in there.

Don't Make a Square Wheel!

This workout is a science—like the law of gravity, it has to work. Bodybuilders have been using it for years. It took them fifty years to perfect it. It's as if they invented the wheel. Don't try to reinvent the wheel. Just because it's taking a little longer for your cart to reach its journey, don't start saying the wheel doesn't work. Don't start trying to reinvent the wheel (jumping to other workouts). You'll make a square wheel. It won't work! Keep going with this workout. The entire community of bodybuilders and I have done all the work for you. Take advantage of it.

Take a before photo. Take one in five weeks and another every five weeks. Send me the photos, even if you don't think you saw any progress. I'll scrutinize them. Include a stamped, self-addressed envelope and I'll comment and encourage you. This works. I know it, but you don't yet. You're just at a sticking point. Your body will break through. You'll see.

What to Do if You Feel Depressed and Just Don't Have the Energy

This can be the hardest time to work out. It isn't so much that your body is too weak to move—it's your mind that's affecting your body, draining it of energy so that you wonder if you could move even if a fire broke out and your life depended upon it.

Negative thinking and discouragement is a sneaky thing. It creeps up on you unawares. Your mind starts telling you, "Oh, what's the point. Look at you, you're so out of shape—the workout you will do today is like a drop in the bucket—it won't make much of a difference. You'll have to work out for years before you see anything, and even then probably nothing will happen. Let's face it—you are too far gone." And you feel too tired to move.

Or you may wake up in the morning and think of working out (that's when you have decided to do it), and say to yourself, "I have a hard life. I get precious little sleep as it is," and you may decide to press the snooze button. Then you may remember the problems in your life and pull the covers over your head and hibernate. "I deserve to sleep another ten minutes," you think. "Nobody will die if I don't work out today," you reason. "And anyway, why punish myself, doesn't the world do that to me enough," you conclude, and you go into a catatonic state, planning to press the snooze button a few more times—until it is safely too late to work out.

Or, you may get home from a hard day at work and think of going straight to the workout area like you usually do, but you think, "I hate my life. All I do is go from one responsibility to another. When am I going to catch a break? When am I going to get a crumb of pleasure. *I'm not working out today.* I'm going to go straight to the refrigerator and get some food and rest my body on the couch while I watch TV."

Or you may have had some bad news today. Your boss refused you a raise, your teenage daughter is pregnant, you found out that your husband or boy-friend is cheating on you, two unexpected bills came in the mail, you just broke a nail. "Are you kidding?" you think. "I'm not working out today. I've got too many problems."

Hello. Why not? Will any of the above improve or change if you don't work out? Of course not. The world will go on exactly like it is, and you will continue to have to deal with the various ups and downs of life, only if you don't work out, you'll continue to be fat, out of shape, and more depressed while you do it. On the other hand, if you overcome your temptation to not work out, and if you continue to do so each time you are tempted to not work out, you will not only feel better about yourself because of the way you will look in a few months, and especially in a year, but you will be able to transfer the success of having transformed your body into successes in other life challenges. Instead of giving up when other things seem impossible, you will go on, fueled by your success in conquering your body problem.

If your boss refused you a raise, he had the power to do that—but why give him the power to come into your home and stop you from working out? You didn't have the omnipotence to stop your daughter from having sex with her boyfriend and becoming pregnant, but you do have the power to work out even though she got pregnant. You didn't have the power to stop your husband or boyfriend from cheating on you—even though you foolishly secretly wonder if it was your fault—but you do have the power to create for yourself a sexy body that will bolster your self-confidence and help you stop obsessing about the way you look, so that you can get on with your life and be the charming, energetic, successful person that you were meant to be. The bills won't get paid any faster if you don't work out, and yes, not working out will not cause your broken nail to grow back. But it will make you feel so good about yourself that things will fall into perspective, and a broken nail will seem the least of your problems.

See how it works. It's a trap: you feel depressed, so you tell yourself, "With all of these problems, the last thing I need to do is work out." Your problems feel like burdens: they physically weigh on you and make you feel weak. "I can't do it," you think. "I'm too tired. I deserve a break." But the moment you realize that it's a trap, and that you don't have to fall into the trap, and that, in fact, *at least your workout is something that you can control*, you do it. You do it and you say, "This one's for me." And in a few minutes, when the endorphins (those enzymes that become activated after five minutes of working out) begin to kick in, and you start feeling that natural high, you begin to think more positive thoughts. You begin to look at the world through sunnier glasses. It happens every time. By the time you finish your workout, it seems as if the sun is peeking out from behind the clouds. You get a second wind about your problems. You can cope. The workout does that. It really does.

What to Do When Something Has Interfered with Your Regular Workout Time, and Now It Is Later in the Day and You Don't Feel Like Working Out

It feels like an imposition. You've got a plan A and a plan B. You've set a regular workout time for yourself, plan A, but you have a plan B at the ready, so that if something happens, you can automatically switch to plan B. For example, plan A was to always work out first thing in the morning, but you overslept that day and have to rush to work; however, you have a plan B where you know you are automatically going to have to work out after the children are in bed.

You know this. But now that it has happened, you just don't want to do it. You resent it. You've gone through your day, come home from work, had dinner with the family, straightened up the house, played with the children and tucked them into bed. Now you want to relax. The last thing you want to do is go to the workout area and work out—even though it will take you only fifteen to thirty minutes to do (depending upon which plan you chose).

"I'll do it tomorrow," you think. "One day won't make a difference." But it will. You see, it's the idea of it. In fact this is a test of will. This is a golden opportunity for you to increase your inner strength, and in turn, your power over your life. By working out when you least feel like it, you put yourself in a permanently stronger position of control in that area. The next time it happens (and it will) it won't be as much of a struggle, and the time after that it will be even easier. In time, it is a very minor twinge of temptation. Before you know it, you are in more and more control of your workout life—and in turn, your life. You are no longer the victim of circumstances.

I remember when I used to run at 4:30 A.M. I didn't know what I was doing then. I thought running was going to get me in shape. Since my job was two hours away, and I had to be there at 7:30, if I wanted to run in the morning, I had to do it at that ungodly hour. Some days it would be snowing. Other days there would be ice on the ground. Some days it would be ten below zero. But I would force myself out there and I would do it. It got to the point where the local police car would look for me each day and wave, and even ask me if I noticed anything suspicious if they happened to be looking for a suspect that day.

"You can't run in the rain," they said. "Why, you'll get yourself soaking wet." So what. I got home drenched, threw my clothing in the washing machine, took a hot shower and felt like a million dollars. "You can't run on ice," they said. "You'll slip and fall and break your back." It doesn't have to happen if you step lightly, and step lightly I did, as I gamboled over the ice like a deer! "You can't run in below-zero weather. It'll destroy your lungs," they argued. Not if you bundle up properly with a mouth protector! And on and on and on. "You can't do it." Really? It depends upon how important it is to you!

Overcome it. That's what I learned to do and that's what I'm asking you to do. Bite the bullet. Suck it up! Just do it!

"Oh, that explains it," you may be thinking. "I see it now, she's a nut. No wonder she expects us to overcome our temptation to not work out. For her, it's easy. She's crazy, no normal person would run on ice in below-zero weather at 4:30 A.M."

Okay. I'll give you that. I was crazy. I would never do now at age fifty-two what I did at thirty. I would never think of running at 4:30 A.M. in below-zero weather on ice now—but I did it because I thought (I now know I was wrong) that it would get me in shape, and even though it didn't get me in shape, I did learn an important lesson from it. I learned that the "impossible" can be achieved, and guess what? I'm asking *you* to do the impossible now. And lucky for you, what I'm asking you to do is not crazy, and it *will* get you in shape.

Your working out first thing in the morning when you could be getting fifteen minutes' extra sleep, or giving up part of your lunch hour at work when you get precious little time for lunch as it is, or working out after the children are asleep when that's the last thing in the world you feel like doing: it may be your equivalent to my running on ice in below-zero weather at 4:30 in the morning. I know that. But by an act of will, because it was important to me, because I wanted it badly enough, I did it—and you can too.

What if You Would Rather Watch TV, Eat, Talk on the Phone, or Have a Drink Than Work Out?

We all have these days. In fact, when I was working two jobs, I had them every single day. I was already getting up at 5:00 A.M. to catch the 6:30 train to work. I wasn't about to get up even one minute earlier to do my workout, so I had to do it when I got home—on the three days I didn't go to my second job, anytime after 4:00 P.M. Every time my train pulled into my home station, my joy of arriving home would be quickly dispelled by the awful reminder that I had to work out. Work out? I didn't want to work out. I wanted to sit in front of the TV and eat and relax. I had had a very hard day on my feet—and commuting a total of four hours. The last thing in the world I wanted to do was work out.

But I wanted the prize, so I knew I had to pay the price. I worked out a system where I allowed myself one hour to watch one of the talk shows, and when the closing music came on, I used that as a signal, like one of Pavlov's dogs. I would march myself straight to my workout area, pick up the dumbbells, and begin. In a few minutes I would be feeling much happier and would in fact be wondering why I had made such a big deal about working out. Mind you, I had to win this battle on a daily basis. But each time I won it, later I would think, "I'm so glad I worked out." And afterward I would have no guilt about relaxing on the couch and reading a book, talking on the phone, or working on some favorite project.

It's the same for all of us. It's the law of inertia. We want to keep doing what we've been doing. We don't want to stir ourselves up to change motion. But I want you to know this. *By an act of will*, you can make that move. You can make a plan and condition yourself to follow through on that plan, and you can do this no matter what your workout time—morning, noon, after work, or late evening. You can be in control if you refuse to give in to the law of inertia.

Sometimes your life will change so that you can squeeze a workout in at lunchtime. I loved when I was able to do that. I discovered a local YMCA that had free weights. I joined and it was well worth it, because it meant that I could get my workout over with during my lunch break, and when I got home I would be free. Every time I was tempted to skip a lunchtime workout, I would remember how happy I would be when I got home and didn't have to work out, and when that thought would come, "You have to work out," how great it felt to say, "Ha ha, no I don't, I already worked out."

If we're going to talk about ideal: to me, the best time to work out is the first thing in the morning, before you even have time to think about it. You can condition yourself to march to the workout area right after you go to the bathroom, brush your teeth, and throw some water on your face. Act like a robot without a mind. Just do it. I used to do that when my schedule allowed, and I loved it. But no matter how life makes us change our ideal plans, we can get used to a new plan if it's important enough, and it *is* important enough. If you think of it this way, instead of resenting the alternate plan and thinking of it as an inconvenience and an imposition, instead of fighting plan B, you'll be thankful that you have it, and instead think of it as a lifesaver that allows you to maintain, in at least one small, but very important area, a certain amount of control over your life.

How to Get Back in the Swing When You've Stopped Working Out for a Few Weeks and Are Too Disgusted with Yourself to Start Again

Forgiveness is the key word here. Why are we so hard on ourselves? If you had a friend who talked to you the way you silently talk to yourself, I bet you would drop that friend in a minute. Think of it. Suppose your friend said to you, "You know you're never going to make it. Here you go again. You started the workout and did great for a week, and then boom! the holidays came along and you stopped completely, and now look at you, fatter than ever, and who are you kidding anyway, did you really think you were suddenly going to get discipline? What a loser you are!"

A friend would never say such things to you. A true friend would say something like, "So what if you weakened for a while. Just start again. We falter and stumble at many things in life, but if we don't give up, if we go back at it with forgiveness for our human frailties, we eventually get on track."

Overcoming and winning works with other things you almost quit. For example, did you ever take a course in school where you were absent for a while and thought of dropping the course, but didn't—and you passed after all? To use another example, women have told me that they went out with a man and then lost touch with him for a while, and when he called after all those weeks, thought of never seeing him again, but did anyway, and ended up marrying that man.

You never know. You just never know. So don't quit just because you took a few weeks off—no matter why you took them off—out of sickness, business, laziness, or whatever. If you give it one more try, the time will come when this workout will be a normal part of your daily routine, like brushing your teeth every morning. You'll just do it!

What to Do When You're Feeling Sore from a Previous Workout, and Are Thinking, "Joyce Is Out of Her Mind, I Can't Work Out Today!"

Remember that five minutes into the workout your muscles will begin to feel better as the blood begins to circulate and act as a massage to your muscles. Remember that if you give in to the temptation to wait it out until the soreness goes away, you will be back to square one and have to start all over with the soreness. Rejoice and be thrilled that you are sore—remember that every single spot that is sore marks the spot, just like a map, where a sexy, shapely, defined muscle is replacing fat and filling in loose, sagging skin.

Remember that if you refuse to give in to this weakness, it will help you to resist giving in to other weaknesses—and the carryover can help you become more successful in anything you try. Repeat my favorite motto: "When the going gets tough, the tough get going." Think about how you will feel about yourself later in the day when you realize that you didn't let the soreness stop you, as opposed to how you will feel when you realize that you buckled under—lay down like a defeated dog, and said, "Take me," to the soreness. Remember that anyone can take the path of least resistance—in fact, every loser in the world does just that. And finally, think of me and bite the bullet, and forge ahead. In short, just do it and tell me about it. Write to me and tell me exactly how you felt and how you worked out in spite of it. I'll be proud of you.

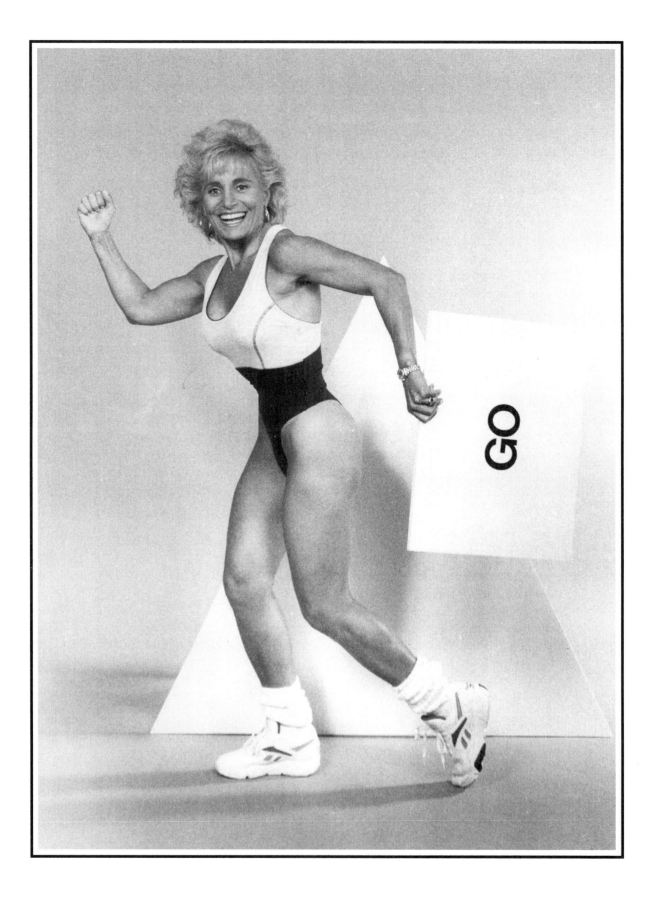

8

THE DEFINITION WORKOUT

The entire workout is found in this chapter. If you are following the fifteen-minute, six-day-a-week plan, you will exercise only the first four body parts on workout day one: chest, triceps, shoulders, and biceps, and the other five body parts, thighs, hips/buttocks, abdominals, back, and calves on workout day two.

If you are following the thirty-minute, three-day-a-week plan, you will of course do the entire workout in one day.

If you are doing the regular workout, do only the first two exercises for each body part. If you're doing the Wonder Woman workout, do only the first three exercises for each body part. If, however, you are doing the Dragon Lady workout, do all four exercises for each body part. As explained in Chapter 6, you will speed-superset all exercises if you are doing the regular or Dragon Lady workouts, and speed-set the odd exercise if you are doing the Wonder Woman workout. You will be reminded of this throughout the exercise instructions.

A WORD ABOUT THE ORDER OF THE EXERCISES

You may notice that the order of exercises in this book is quite different from that of any other book I've written. There is a reason for this: prevention of fatigue. Since this is a very intense workout, it is necessary to separate the exercising of "helping" body parts where possible. For example, instead of asking you to exercise your shoulders right after your chest (shoulders do some work while you are exercising the chest), or biceps (which are slightly involved in the chest exercises), I ask you to work your triceps muscles, which are barely involved in chest work. After you exercise your triceps, instead of asking you to exercise your biceps (which work in opposition to the triceps), I ask you to exercise the shoulders, which are not involved in the triceps movement. Finally, you exercise your biceps—which are not involved in shoulder movement. Biceps are your last body part for workout day one if you are doing the fifteen-minute workout.

Thighs are exercised before any other lower body part because this body part requires the most effort of all lower body parts and it's a good idea to give this area your first thrust of energy. Hips/buttocks, although closely connected to the thighs, are exercised next because they require no weights, and require so much less effort than do the thighs that you have a chance to, in a way, catch your breath. Abdominals are next in line because they take a lot of effort—yet you don't want to save them for last or you will dread doing them and may even be tempted to skip them. Your back is next because it is always relaxing to exercise the back—a perfect way to approach the end of your workout. And calves are last because they are so easy to exercise that they almost don't count in terms of energy expenditure. No matter how tired you are, you won't be tempted to skip calves. Comparatively speaking, you could exercise your calves in your sleep.

READ THE EXERCISE INSTRUCTIONS!

I realize that you will be looking at the photographs as opposed to reading the exercise instructions when doing your workout, but you must read the exercise instructions with a pen or pencil in hand the first time you work out—underlining significant points that you think you will need to remember. Pay special attention to the "Beware" section.

SETS, REPETITIONS, AND WEIGHTS: A QUICK REVIEW

Chest, triceps, shoulders, biceps, thighs, back, and calves will require the full pyramid system as follows:

Set 1: twelve repetitions, one-pound dumbbells
Set 2: ten repetitions, two-pound dumbbells
Set 3: eight repetitions, three-pound dumbbells
Set 4: ten repetitions, two-pound dumbbells
Set 5: twelve repetitions, one-pound dumbbells

Reminder: the pounds in reference to dumbbells *always* refer to each dumbbell. Also, the pounds used in the above example will be higher throughout as you eventually become stronger and increase your weights. In other words, instead of using one-, two-, and three-pound dumbbells, you will eventually use two-, three-, and five-pound dumbbells, and eventually, three-, five-, and eight-pound dumbbells, and so on. In fact, if you see that the very light weight dumbbells are too easy to begin with, you may start with the higher weights. (See page 78 for review.)

Hips/buttocks and abdominal exercises require no weights, so of course you will not use the pyramid system for those body parts (how can you pyramid when there is no weight to pyramid?). Instead, you will simply do fifteen repetitions for all five sets of these exercises. (See page 80 for a discussion as to why this is so.)

CHEST ROUTINE
Superset: Flat Flye with Flat Press

(Wonder Woman routine: add and speed-set incline flye. Dragon Lady routine: add and speed-superset incline flye with incline press.)

   Note: I am using a "step" that is ten inches off the ground in place of a bench, so whenever I say "bench," I mean bench or step.

1. Flat Flye

This exercise develops, shapes, strengthens, and defines the entire chest (pectoral) area.

Position: Lie with your back flat against the bench, holding a dumbbell in each hand. (You have the option of placing your feet on the bench or on the floor.) With your palms facing each other, extend your arms straight up so that the dumbbells are touching in the center of your body. Do not lock your elbows.

Movement: With your elbows slightly bent, extend your arms outward and downward in a semicircle until you feel a complete stretch in your pectoral muscles. Flexing your pectoral muscles, return to start position and repeat the movement until you have completed your set.

   Without resting, proceed to the other exercise in this superset, the flat press.

Beware: Don't hold your breath. Breathe naturally. Don't swing the dumbbells wildly. Maintain control. Keep your elbows slightly bent throughout the movement. Think of your arms as slightly curved steel bars that cannot be bent. Keep your back flat on the bench as you work.

Machines, etc.: Pec Deck Machine.

SETS, REPETITIONS, WEIGHTS

Set 1: 12 reps flat flye + 12 reps flat press, 1-pound dumbbells
Set 2: 10 reps flat flye + 10 reps flat press, 2-pound dumbbells
Set 3: 8 reps flat flye + 8 reps flat press, 3-pound dumbbells
Set 4: 10 reps flat flye + 10 reps flat press, 2-pound dumbbells
Set 5: 12 reps flat flye + 12 reps flat press, 1-pound dumbbells

Rest 15 seconds and move to the next exercise.

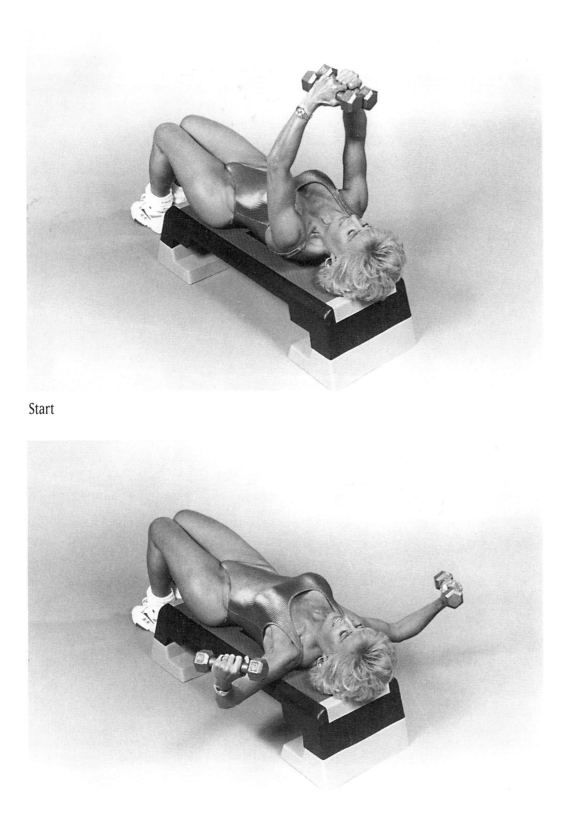

Start

Finish

2. Flat Press

This exercise develops, shapes, strengthens, and defines the entire chest (pectoral) area.

Position: Lie on a flat exercise bench with a dumbbell held in each hand, palms facing upward, and with the inner edge of the dumbbells touching your upper chest area.

Movement: Flexing your chest muscles as you go, extend your arms upward until your elbows are nearly locked. The dumbbells should be in line with your upper chest in this fully extended position. Willfully flex your pectoral muscles and return to start position. Feel the stretch in your pectoral muscles and repeat the movement until you have completed your set.

Without resting, perform your second through fifth sets of this exercise combination—the flat flye and the flat press.

Beware: In order to get a full stretch in your chest, be sure to extend your elbows fully downward on the down movement. Keep your mind focused on your chest muscles throughout the exercise.

Machines, etc.: You may use any bench press machine in place of this exercise.

SETS, REPETITIONS, WEIGHTS

(same as page 116—repeated here for review):

Set 1: 12 reps flat flye + 12 reps flat press, 1-pound dumbbells
Set 2: 10 reps flat flye + 10 reps flat press, 2-pound dumbbells
Set 3: 8 reps flat flye + 8 reps flat press, 3-pound dumbbells
Set 4: 10 reps flat flye + 10 reps flat press, 2-pound dumbbells
Set 5: 12 reps flat flye + 12 reps flat press, 1-pound dumbbells

Rest 15 seconds and move to the next exercise.

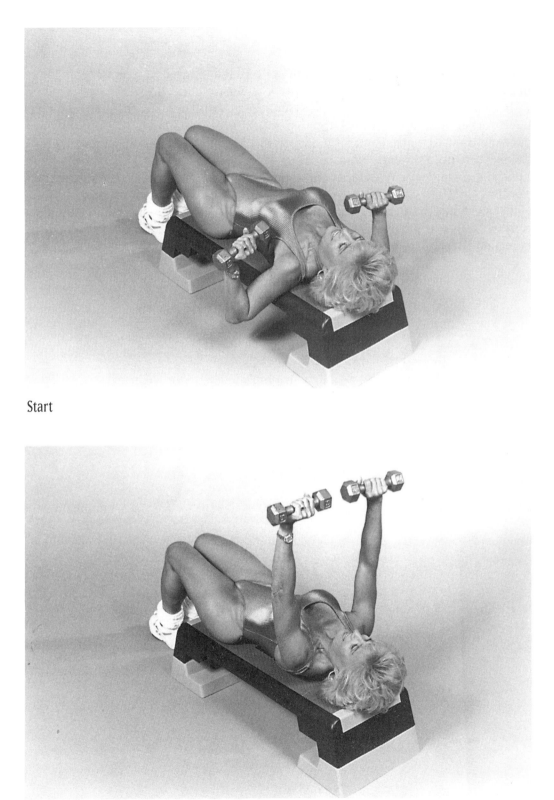

Start

Finish

3. Incline Flye

(For Wonder Woman routine: add and speed-set incline flye. For Dragon Lady routine: add and speed-superset incline flye with incline press.)

This exercise develops, shapes, strengthens, and defines the entire chest (pectoral) area, especially the upper pectoral area.

Follow the instructions exactly as you did for the flat flye, only this time do the exercise on an incline bench.

If you are doing the Wonder Woman workout, you will have speed-setted this exercise, and then you will move on to your next body part, your triceps routine. If you are doing the Dragon Lady routine, you will have speed-supersetted this exercise with the incline press. You will then rest 15 seconds and proceed to your next body part, the triceps.

SETS, REPETITIONS, WEIGHTS

(Wonder Woman routine):

Set 1: 12 reps incline flye, 1-pound dumbbells
Set 2: 10 reps incline flye, 2-pound dumbbells
Set 3: 8 reps incline flye, 3-pound dumbbells
Set 4: 10 reps incline flye, 2-pound dumbbells
Set 5: 12 reps incline flye, 1-pound dumbbells

Rest 15 seconds and move to the next exercise.

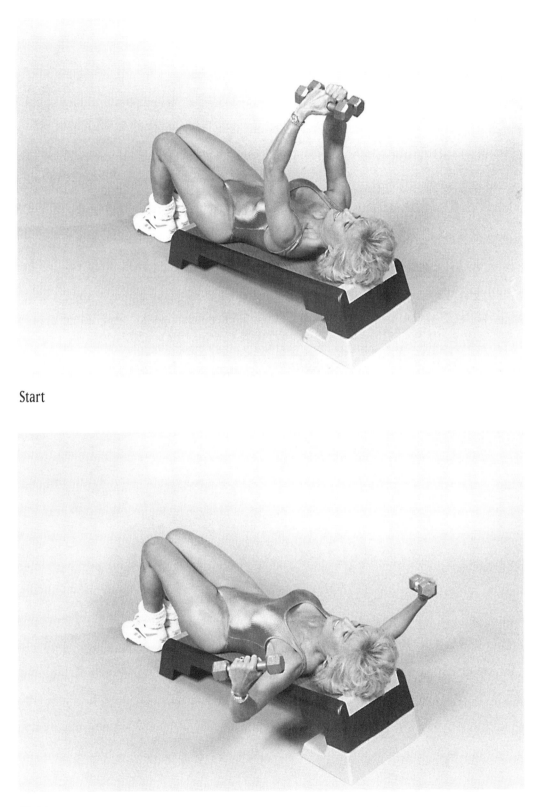

Start

Finish

4. Incline Press

(For Dragon Lady routine: speed-superset this exercise with the incline flye.)

This exercise develops, shapes, strengthens, and defines the entire chest (pectoral) area, especially the upper pectoral area.

Follow the instructions exactly as you did for the flat press, only this time do the exercise on an incline bench.

Without resting, perform your second through fifth sets of this exercise combination—the incline flye and the incline press, then rest 15 seconds and proceed to the next body part, the triceps.

SETS, REPETITIONS, WEIGHTS

(Dragon Lady routine):

Set 1: 12 reps incline flye + 12 reps incline press, 1-pound dumbbells
Set 2: 10 reps incline flye + 10 reps incline press, 2-pound dumbbells
Set 3: 8 reps incline flye + 8 reps incline press, 3-pound dumbbells
Set 4: 10 reps incline flye + 10 reps incline press, 2-pound dumbbells
Set 5: 12 reps incline flye + 12 reps incline press, 1-pound dumbbells

Rest 15 seconds and move to the next exercise.

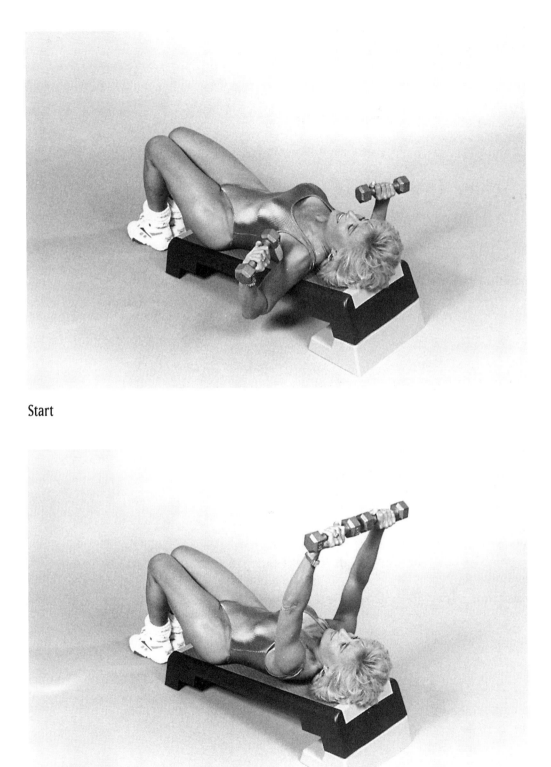

Start

Finish

TRICEPS ROUTINE
Superset: Seated Overhead Press with Close Bench Press

(Wonder Woman routine: add and speed-set simultaneous kickback. Dragon Lady routine: add and speed-superset simultaneous kickback with lying extension.)

I. Seated Overhead Press

This exercise develops, shapes, strengthens, and defines the entire triceps, especially the inside and rear heads of this muscle.

Position: Grasp a dumbbell with both hands with an overhead grip, holding it on either side of the ball shape. Sit on a flat bench or chair, and raise the dumbbell straight up, locking your elbows and keeping your biceps close to your ears.

Movement: Keeping your biceps close to your head, and your elbows stationary, lower the dumbbell in an arclike movement by letting your arms descend behind you. Feel a full stretch in your triceps muscle, and without resting, and flexing your triceps muscles as you go, return to start position. Willfully flex your triceps muscle and repeat the movement until you have completed your set.

Without resting, proceed to the other exercise in this superset, the close bench press.

Beware: Your upper arms must remain close to your head throughout the movement. Don't hold your breath. Breathe naturally.

Machines, etc: You may use either a regular barbell or an "Ez Curl bar" to perform this exercise.

SETS, REPETITIONS, WEIGHTS

Set 1: 12 reps seated overhead press + 12 reps close bench press, 1-pound dumbbells

Set 2: 10 reps seated overhead press + 10 reps close bench press, 2-pound dumbbells

Set 3: 8 reps seated overhead press + 8 reps close bench press, 3-pound dumbbells

Set 4: 10 reps seated overhead press + 10 reps close bench press, 2-pound dumbbells

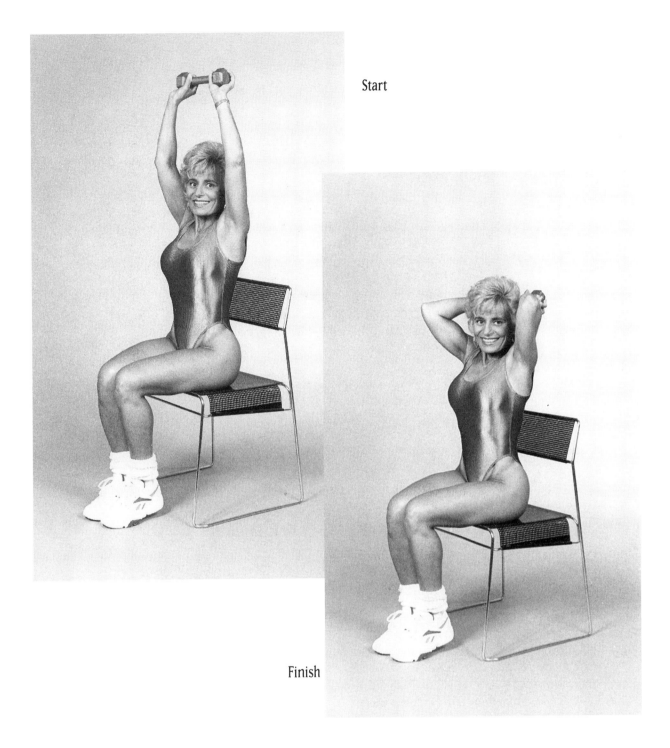

Start

Finish

Set 5: 12 reps seated overhead press + 12 reps close bench press, 1-pound dumbbells

Rest 15 seconds and move to the next exercise.

2. Close Bench Press

This exercise develops, shapes, strengthens, and defines the entire triceps.

Position: Lie on a flat exercise bench and grip a dumbbell with both hands, palms facing upward. Hold the dumbbell close to the center of your chest, and grip the ball at the end of the dumbbell with each hand.

Movement: Flexing your triceps muscles as you go, and keeping your elbows close to your body, raise your arms upward until they are fully extended. Willfully flex your triceps and, continuing to keep your elbows close to your body, return to start position. Feel the stretch in your triceps muscle and repeat the movement until you have completed your set.

Without resting, perform your second through fifth sets of this exercise combination—the seated overhead press and the close bench press.

Beware: In order to make sure that your triceps do the work, it is mandatory that you keep your upper arms close to your body throughout the exercise.

Machines, etc.: You may use a regular barbell for this exercise.

SETS, REPETITIONS, WEIGHTS

(same as pages 124–125—repeated here for review):

Set 1: 12 reps seated overhead press + 12 reps close bench press, 1-pound dumbbells

Set 2: 10 reps seated overhead press + 10 reps close bench press, 2-pound dumbbells

Set 3: 8 reps seated overhead press + 8 reps close bench press, 3-pound dumbbells

Set 4: 10 reps seated overhead press + 10 reps close bench press, 2-pound dumbbells

Set 5: 12 reps seated overhead press + 12 reps close bench press, 1-pound dumbbells

Rest 15 seconds and move to the next exercise.

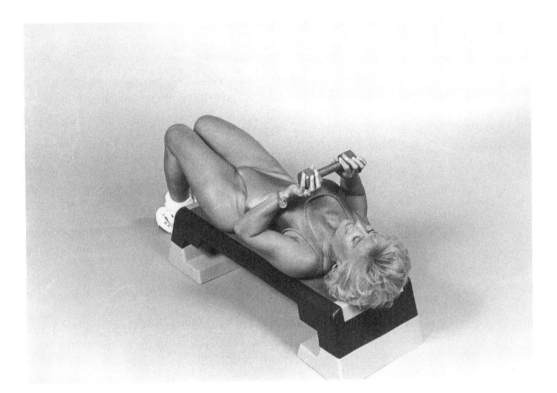

Start

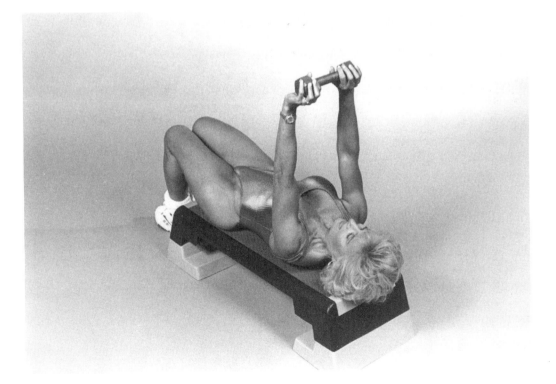

Finish

3. Simultaneous Kickback

(For Wonder Woman routine: add and speed-set simultaneous kickback. For Dragon Lady routine: add and speed-superset simultaneous kickback with lying extension.)

This exercise develops, shapes, strengthens, and defines the entire triceps.

Position: Stand with your feet together, bending at the waist and at the knees, and hold a dumbbell in each hand, palms facing your body. Bend your arm at the elbows so that your forearms are nearly parallel to the floor and your elbows are touching your waist.

Movement: Keeping your upper arms close to your body, and flexing your triceps as you go, extend your arms back as far as possible, and willfully flex your triceps muscles.

Return to start position and feel the stretch in your triceps muscle. Without resting, repeat the movement until you have completed your set. If you are on the Wonder Woman routine, proceed to the next body part, the shoulders. If you are on the Dragon Lady routine you will speed-superset this exercise with the other exercise in this superset, the lying extension.

Beware: Keep your upper arms close to your body throughout the exercise. Don't jerk the dumbbells back. Control your movements. Don't hold your breath. Breathe naturally.

Machines, etc.: You may perform this exercise with a curved triceps pulldown bar, using any machine pulley device.

SETS, REPETITIONS, WEIGHTS

(Wonder Woman routine):

Set 1: 12 reps simultaneous kickback, 1-pound dumbbells
Set 2: 10 reps simultaneous kickback, 2-pound dumbbells
Set 3: 8 reps simultaneous kickback, 3-pound dumbbells
Set 4: 10 reps simultaneous kickback, 2-pound dumbbells
Set 5: 12 reps simultaneous kickback, 1-pound dumbbells

Rest 15 seconds and move to the next exercise.

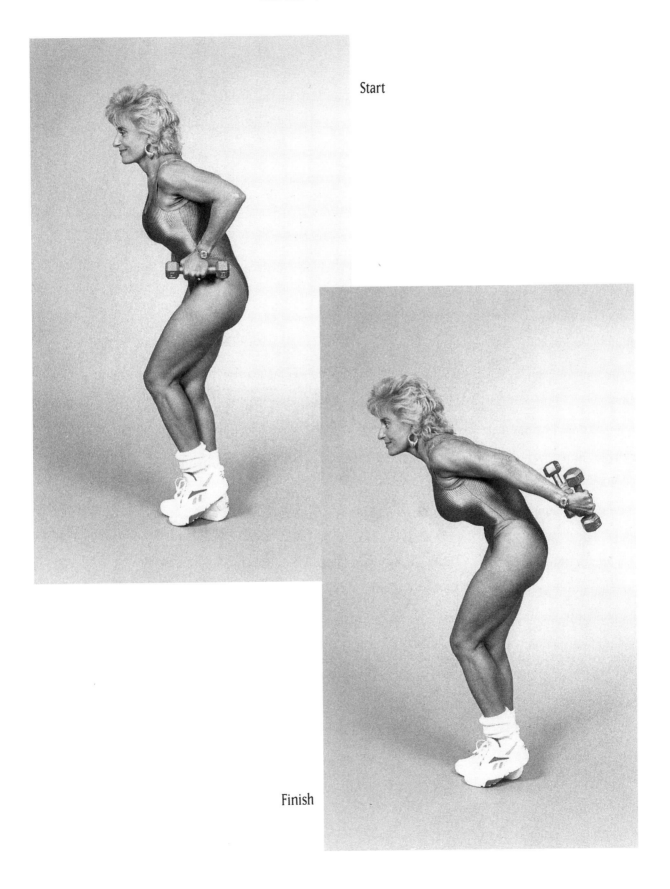

Start

Finish

4. Lying Extension

(For Dragon Lady routine: speed-superset this exercise with simultaneous kick-back.)

This exercise develops, shapes, strengthens, and defines the entire triceps muscle, especially the outer triceps area.

Position: Lie on a flat exercise bench with your knees bent, and the soles of your feet flat on the bench, holding a dumbbell in each hand, palms facing each other. Extend your arms straight up so that the dumbbells are centered above each pectoral muscle.

Movement: Keeping your elbows steady and as stationary as possible, bending at the elbows, simultaneously lower the dumbbells until they reach your shoulders. Feel the stretch in your triceps muscles, and flexing your triceps as you go, return to start position. Willfully flex your triceps, and repeat the movement until you have completed your set.

Without resting, perform your second through fifth sets of this exercise combination—the simultaneous kickback and the lying dumbbell extension. Rest 15 seconds and then proceed to the next body part, the shoulders.

Beware: Keep your elbows in line with your body throughout the movement.

Machines, etc.: You may use any triceps machine in place of this exercise.

SETS, REPETITIONS, WEIGHTS

(Dragon Lady routine):

Set 1: 12 reps simultaneous kickback + 12 reps lying extension, 1-pound dumbbells

Set 2: 10 reps simultaneous kickback + 10 reps lying extension, 2-pound dumbbells

Set 3: 8 reps simultaneous kickback + 8 reps lying extension, 3-pound dumbbells

Set 4: 10 reps simultaneous kickback + 10 reps lying extension, 2-pound dumbbells

Set 5: 12 reps simultaneous kickback + 12 reps lying extension, 1-pound dumbbells

Rest 15 seconds and move to the next exercise.

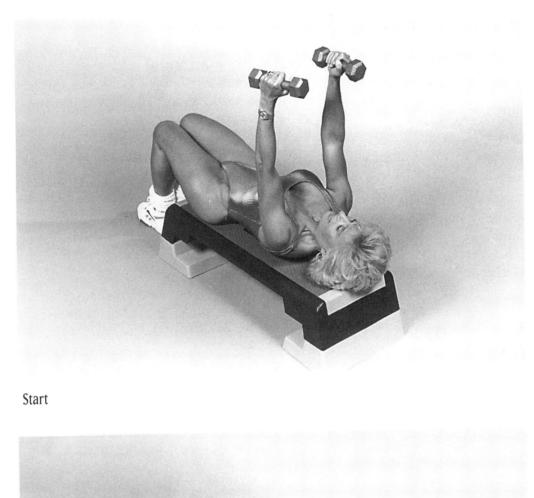

Start

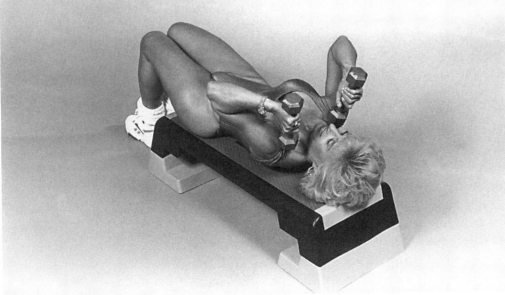

Finish

SHOULDERS ROUTINE
Superset: Reverse Overhead Lateral with Bent Lateral

(Wonder Woman routine: add and speed-set side lateral. Dragon Lady routine: add and speed-superset side lateral with alternate shoulder press.)

I. Reverse Overhead Dumbbell Lateral

This exercise develops, shapes, strengthens, and defines the entire shoulder (deltoid) muscle, especially the front area, and helps to develop the trapezius muscles.

Position: Stand with your feet a natural width apart with a dumbbell in each hand, palms held upward. Extend your arms out to either side so that they are parallel to the floor. Curl your wrists upward and bend your elbows slightly.

Movement: Raise your arms up until the dumbbells touch over your head. Your elbows should remain slightly bent at the top position. Feel the stretch in your shoulder muscles. Return to start position and willfully flex your shoulder muscles. Repeat the movement until you have completed your set.

Without resting, proceed to the other exercise in this superset, the bent lateral.

Beware: Don't let your arms nearly drop to start position. Maintain control of the dumbbells at all times. Don't hold your breath. Breathe naturally.

Machines, etc.: You may substitute this exercise for any machine shoulder exercise, since there is no exact machine substitute.

SETS, REPETITIONS, WEIGHTS

Set 1: 12 reps reverse overhead lateral + 12 reps bent lateral, 1-pound dumbbells
Set 2: 10 reps reverse overhead lateral + 10 reps bent lateral, 2-pound dumbbells
Set 3: 8 reps reverse overhead lateral + 8 reps bent lateral, 3-pound dumbbells
Set 4: 10 reps reverse overhead lateral + 10 reps bent lateral, 2-pound dumbbells
Set 5: 12 reps reverse overhead lateral + 12 reps bent lateral, 1-pound dumbbells

Rest 15 seconds and move to the next exercise.

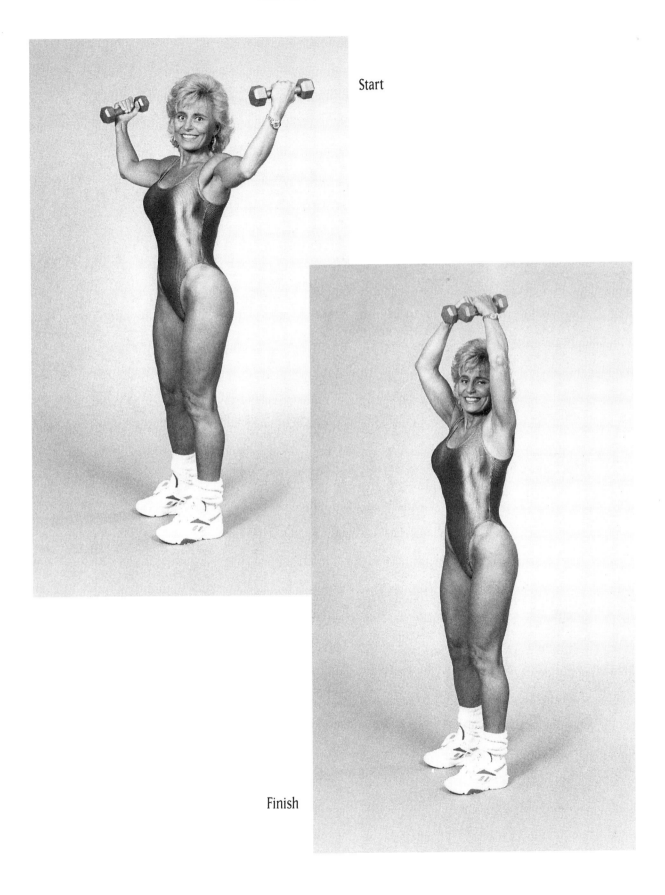

Start

Finish

2. Bent Lateral

This exercise develops, shapes, strengthens, and defines the rear and side shoulder (deltoid) muscles.

Position: Stand with your feet together, holding a dumbbell in each hand, with palms facing each other. Bend over until your upper body is parallel to the floor and extend your arms straight down in front of you in the center of your body. Let the ends of the dumbbells touch each other at about knee height.

Movement: Keeping your wrists slightly bent, and flexing your side and rear shoulder muscles as you go, extend your arms outward until your arms are almost parallel to the floor. Willfully flex your shoulder muscles and return to start. Feel the stretch in your shoulder muscles and repeat the movement until you have completed your set.

Without resting, perform your second through fifth sets of this exercise combination—the reverse overhead lateral and the bent lateral.

Beware: Keep your upper body (torso) parallel to the floor throughout the movement.

Machines, etc.: You may perform this exercise using any spaced-apart floor pulley machine.

SETS, REPETITIONS, WEIGHTS

(same as page 132—repeated here for review):

Set 1: 12 reps reverse overhead lateral + 12 reps bent lateral, 1-pound dumbbells
Set 2: 10 reps reverse overhead lateral + 10 reps bent lateral, 2-pound dumbbells
Set 3: 8 reps reverse overhead lateral + 8 reps bent lateral, 3-pound dumbbells
Set 4: 10 reps reverse overhead lateral + 10 reps bent lateral, 2-pound dumbbells
Set 5: 12 reps reverse overhead lateral + 12 reps bent lateral, 1-pound dumbbells

Rest 15 seconds and move to the next exercise.

Start

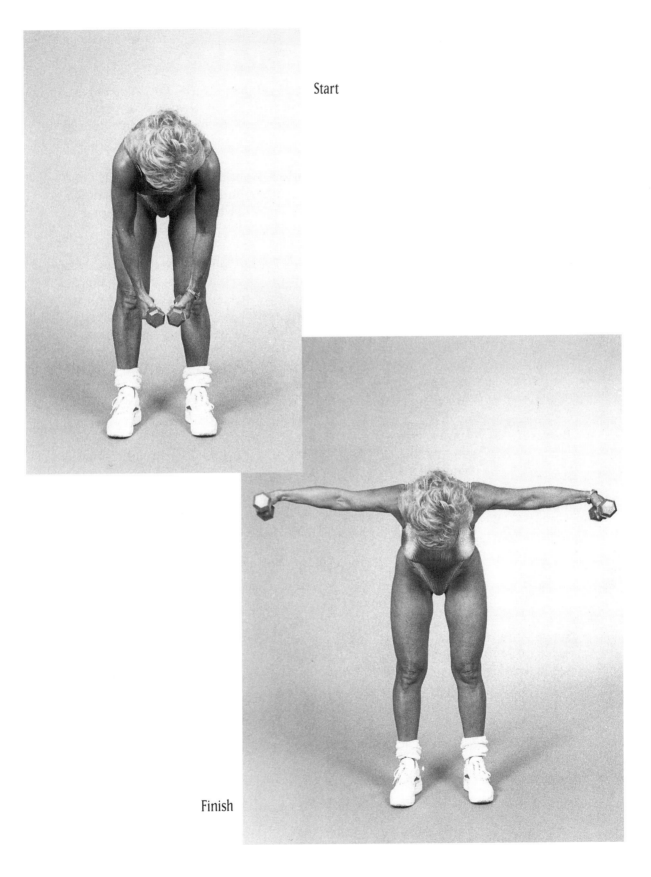

Finish

3. Side Lateral

(For Wonder Woman routine: add and speed-set side lateral. For Dragon Lady routine: add and speed-superset side lateral with alternate shoulder press.)

This exercise develops, shapes, strengthens, and defines the entire deltoid muscle, especially the medial area.

Position: Stand with your feet together. Hold a dumbbell in each hand with your palms facing each other, and extend your arms downward letting the dumbbells touch at the ends in the center of your body.

Movement: Flexing your shoulder muscles as you go, extend your arms upward and outward until the dumbbells are slightly higher than shoulder height. Willfully flex your shoulders and return to start position. Feel the stretch in your shoulder muscles and repeat the movement until you have completed your set.

If you are on the Wonder Woman routine, proceed to the next body part, the biceps. If you are on the Dragon Lady routine, you will speed-superset this exercise with the other exercise in this superset, the alternate shoulder press.

Beware: Don't swing the dumbbells out and up. Use controlled movements, but do keep it moving. Don't hold your breath. Breathe naturally.

Machines, etc.: You may perform this exercise on any shoulder side-lateral machine.

SETS, REPETITIONS, WEIGHTS

(Wonder Woman routine):

Set 1: 12 reps side lateral, 1-pound dumbbells
Set 2: 10 reps side lateral, 2-pound dumbbells
Set 3: 8 reps side lateral, 3-pound dumbbells
Set 4: 10 reps side lateral, 2-pound dumbbells
Set 5: 12 reps side lateral, 1-pound dumbbells.

Rest 15 seconds and move to the next exercise.

Start

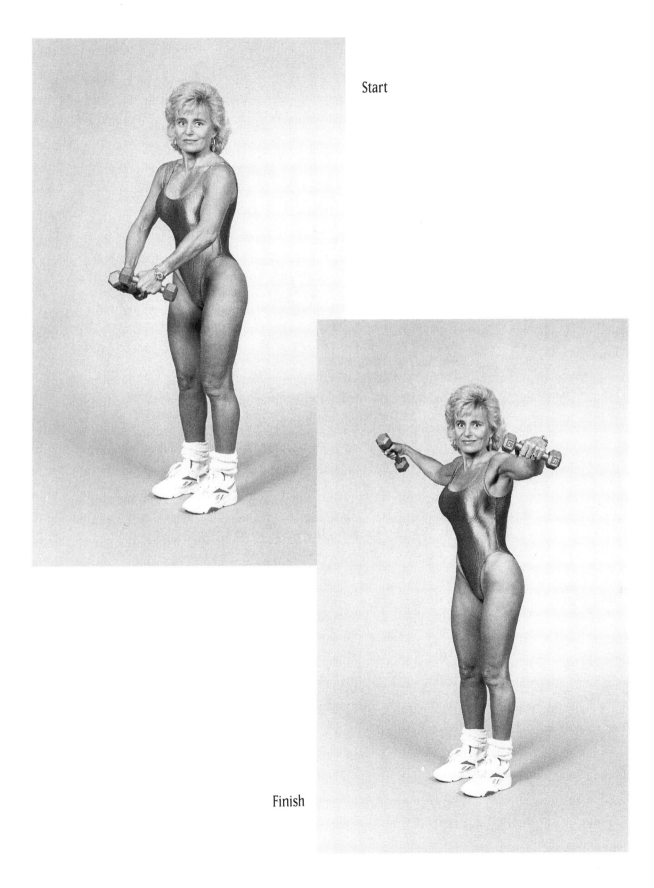

Finish

137

4. Alternate Shoulder Press

(For Dragon Lady routine: speed-superset this exercise with side lateral.)

This exercise develops, shapes, strengthens, and defines the entire shoulder muscle, especially the front area of this muscle.

Position: Stand with your feet together or in a natural position, holding a dumbbell in each hand at shoulder height, with your palms facing away from your body.

Movement: Raise your right arm upward until it is fully extended. While returning your right arm to the start position, begin raising your left arm upward until it is fully extended, while at the same time lowering your right arm. Continue this alternate up-and-down movement until you have completed your set.

Without resting, perform your second through fifth sets of this exercise combination—the side lateral and the alternate shoulder press. Rest 15 seconds and then proceed to the next body part, the biceps.

Beware: Keep your upper body steady as you work. Remember to flex your shoulder muscle on each upward movement, and to feel the stretch on each down position.

Machines, etc.: You may use any shoulder press machine in place of this exercise.

SETS, REPETITIONS, WEIGHTS

(Dragon Lady routine):

Set 1: 12 reps side lateral + 12 reps alternate shoulder press, 1-pound dumbbells
Set 2: 10 reps side lateral + 10 reps alternate shoulder press, 2-pound dumbbells
Set 3: 8 reps side lateral + 8 reps alternate shoulder press, 3-pound dumbbells
Set 4: 10 reps side lateral + 10 reps alternate shoulder press, 2-pound dumbbells
Set 5: 12 reps side lateral + 12 reps alternate shoulder press, 1-pound dumbbells

Rest 15 seconds and move to the next exercise.

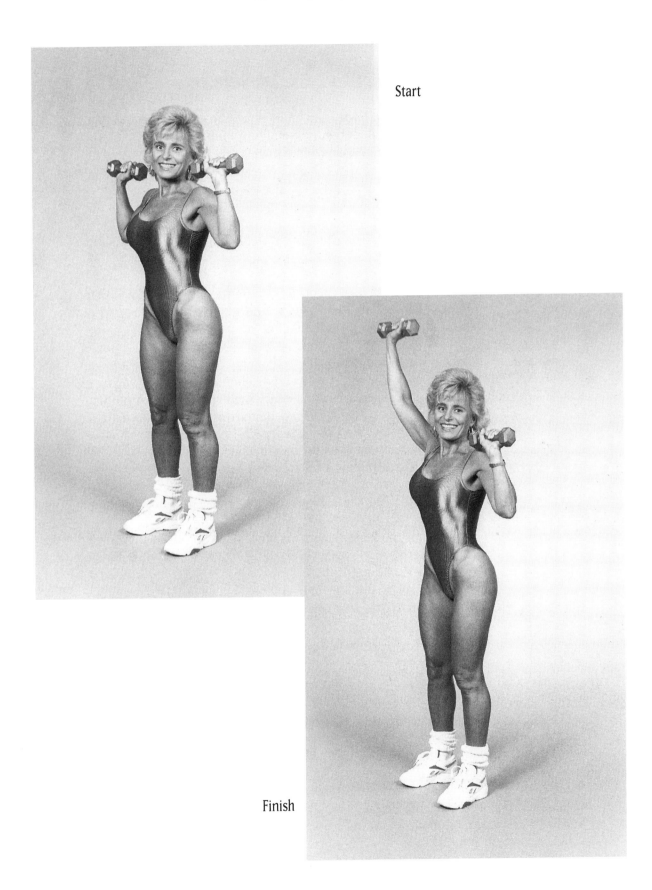

Start

Finish

BICEPS ROUTINE
Superset: Simultaneous Standing Curl with Alternate Reverse Curl

(Wonder Woman routine: add and speed-set lying simultaneous flat-bench curl. Dragon Lady routine: add and speed-superset lying simultaneous flat bench curl with lying alternate flat bench hammer curl.)

1. Simultaneous Standing Curl

This exercise develops, shapes, strengthens, and defines the entire biceps muscle, and helps to strengthen the forearm.

Position: Stand with your feet together or a natural width apart with a dumbbell in each hand. Place your arms at your sides and hold the dumbbells with palms facing your body.

Movement: Flexing your biceps muscles as you go, and keeping your arms close to your body and your wrists slightly curled upward, curl your arms upward simultaneously while turning your palms to face your shoulders until you cannot curl them any further. Willfully flex your biceps muscles and return to start position. Feel the stretch in your biceps muscles and repeat the movement until you have completed your set.

Without resting, proceed to the other exercise in this superset, the alternate reverse curl.

Beware: Don't rock back and forth as you work. Your body should remain stationary—only your arms are moving. Don't hold your breath. Breathe naturally.

Machines, etc.: You may perform this exercise on any biceps curl machine.

SETS, REPETITIONS, WEIGHTS

Set 1: 12 reps simultaneous standing curl + 12 reps alternate reverse curl, 1-pound dumbbells

Set 2: 10 reps simultaneous standing curl + 10 reps alternate reverse curl, 2-pound dumbbells

Set 3: 8 reps simultaneous standing curl + 8 reps alternate reverse curl, 3-pound dumbbells

Set 4: 10 reps simultaneous standing curl + 10 reps alternate reverse curl, 2-pound dumbbells

Set 5: 12 reps simultaneous standing curl + 12 reps alternate reverse curl, 1-pound dumbbells

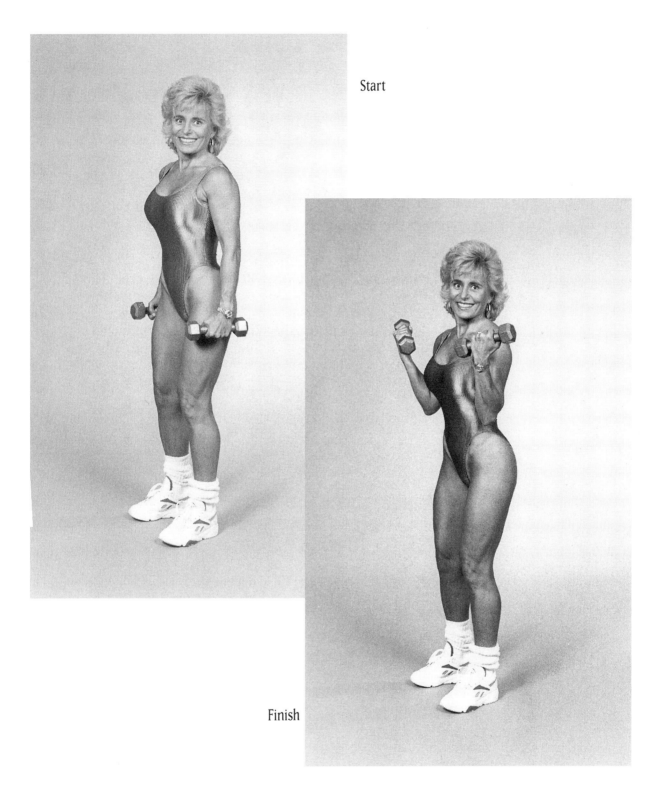

Start

Finish

Rest 15 seconds and move to the next exercise if you are doing the 30-minute workout. Stop here if you are doing the 15-minute workout.

2. Alternate Reverse Curl

This exercise develops, shapes, strengthens, and defines the entire biceps area, especially the outer area, and helps to develop the forearms.

Position: Stand with your feet together or a natural width apart, with a dumbbell in each hand, palms facing your body. Place your arms straight down at your sides, but slightly in front of you.

Movement: Keeping your upper arms as close to your body as you can, curl your right arm up until it cannot go any further. As you begin to allow your right arm to return to start position, begin to curl your left arm upward. As your left arm reaches its highest position, your right arm will be down at your side, at start position. Continue this alternate curling movement until you have completed your set.

Without resting, perform your second through fifth sets of this exercise combination—the simultaneous standing curl and the alternate reverse curl. If you are doing the 15-minute split routine, stop here. Otherwise, rest 15 seconds and move to the next body part, the thighs.

Beware: Remember to flex your biceps on the up movement and to feel the stretch on the down movement. Keep your elbows close to your body throughout the exercise.

Machines, etc.: You may perform this exercise on any forearm machine.

SETS, REPETITIONS, WEIGHTS

(same as page 140—repeated here for review):

Set 1: 12 reps simultaneous standing curl + 12 reps alternate reverse curl, 1-pound dumbbells

Set 2: 10 reps simultaneous standing curl + 10 reps alternate reverse curl, 2-pound dumbbells

Set 3: 8 reps simultaneous standing curl + 8 reps alternate reverse curl, 3-pound dumbbells

Set 4: 10 reps simultaneous standing curl + 10 reps alternate reverse curl, 2-pound dumbbells

Set 5: 12 reps simultaneous standing curl + 12 reps alternate reverse curl, 1-pound dumbbells

Rest 15 seconds and move to the next exercise if you are doing the 30-minute workout. Stop here if you are doing the 15-minute workout.

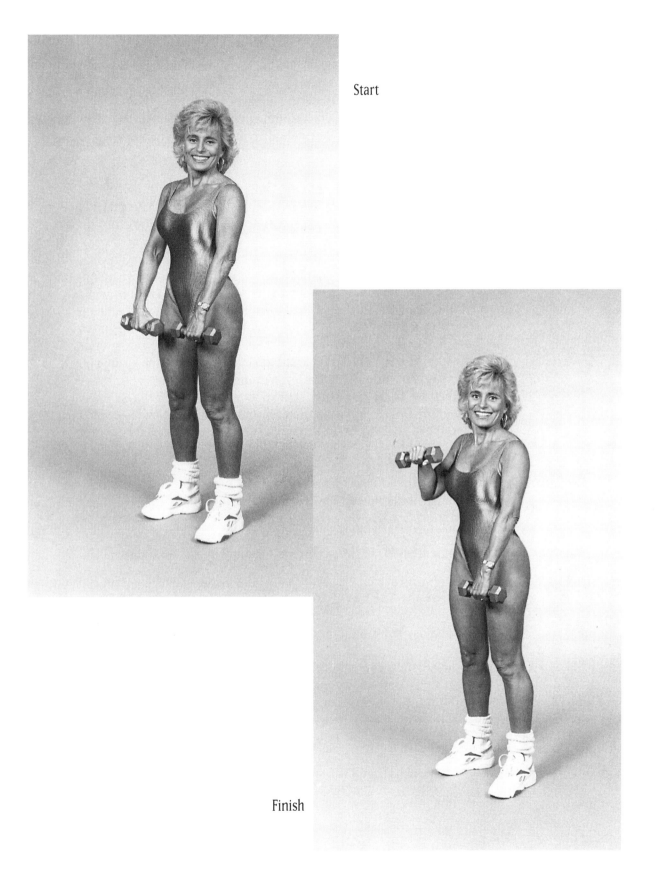

Start

Finish

3. Lying Simultaneous Flat-Bench Curl

(For Wonder Woman routine: add and speed-set lying simultaneous flat-bench curl. For Dragon Lady routine: add and speed-superset lying simultaneous flat bench curl with lying alternate flat-bench hammer curl.)

This exercise develops, strengthens, and defines the entire biceps area, especially the peak.

Position: With a dumbbell in each hand, palms facing your body, lie on your back on a flat exercise bench. Let your arms extend fully downward so that you can feel the stretch in your biceps muscles.

Movement: Twisting your wrists so that your palms face upward, and flexing your biceps muscles as you go, curl your arms upward until you cannot go any further. (The dumbbells should be nearly touching your shoulders.) Willfully flex your biceps muscles and return to start position. Feel the stretch in your biceps and repeat the movement until you have completed your set.

If you are using the Wonder Woman routine, proceed to the next body part, the thighs. If you are on the Dragon Lady routine, you will speed-superset this exercise with the other exercise in this superset, the lying alternate flat-bench hammer curl.

Beware: Don't let the dumbbells nearly drop down to start position. Maintain control. Don't let your body rise from the bench. Don't hold your breath. Breathe naturally.

Machines, etc.: You may perform this exercise on any biceps machine.

SETS, REPETITIONS, WEIGHTS

(Wonder Woman routine):

Set 1: 12 reps lying simultaneous flat-bench curl, 1-pound dumbbells
Set 2: 10 reps lying simultaneous flat-bench curl, 2-pound dumbbells
Set 3: 8 reps lying simultaneous flat-bench curl, 3-pound dumbbells
Set 4: 10 reps lying simultaneous flat-bench curl, 2-pound dumbbells
Set 5: 12 reps lying simultaneous flat-bench curl, 1-pound dumbbells

Rest 15 seconds and move to the next exercise if you are doing the 30-minute workout. Stop here if you are doing the 15-minute workout.

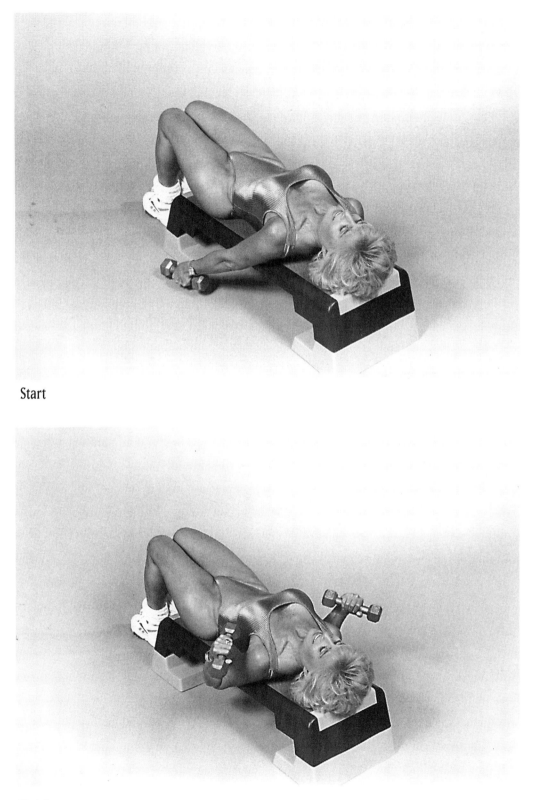

Start

Finish

4. Lying Alternate Flat-Bench Hammer Curl

(For Dragon Lady routine: speed-superset this exercise with lying simultaneous flat-bench curl.)

This exercise develops, shapes, strengthens, and defines the entire biceps area and helps to develop the forearms.

Position: With a dumbbell in each hand, palms facing your body, lie on your back on a flat exercise bench. Let your arms extend fully downward so you can feel the full stretch in your biceps. (The dumbbells will be in the "ready-to-hammer" position.)

Movement: Flexing your biceps as you go, and keeping the dumbbell in the hammer position, and close to your body, curl your right arm up until it cannot go any further. At this point begin to curl your left arm up, and at the same time, to lower your right arm to start position. When your right arm reaches start (down) position, your left arm will be in its highest position. Continue this alternate hammer movement until you have completed your set.

Without resting, perform your second through fifth sets of this exercise combination—the lying simultaneous flat-bench curl and the lying alternate flat-bench hammer curl. If you are doing the 15-minute split routine, stop here. Otherwise, rest 15 seconds and proceed to the next body part, the thighs.

Beware: Don't allow your elbows to wander away from your body. Keep them close to your sides. Don't allow your back to rise from the bench. Remember to flex your biceps on each up movement and to feel the stretch in your biceps on each down movement.

Machines, etc.: You may use any biceps machine in place of this exercise.

SETS, REPETITIONS, WEIGHTS

(Dragon Lady routine):

Set 1: 12 reps lying simultaneous flat-bench curl + 12 reps lying alternate flat-bench hammer curl, 1-pound dumbbells

Set 2: 10 reps lying simultaneous flat-bench curl + 10 reps lying alternate flat-bench hammer curl, 2-pound dumbbells

Set 3: 8 reps lying simultaneous flat-bench curl + 8 reps lying alternate flat-bench hammer curl, 3-pound dumbbells

Set 4: 10 reps lying simultaneous flat-bench curl + 10 reps lying alternate flat-bench hammer curl, 2-pound dumbbells

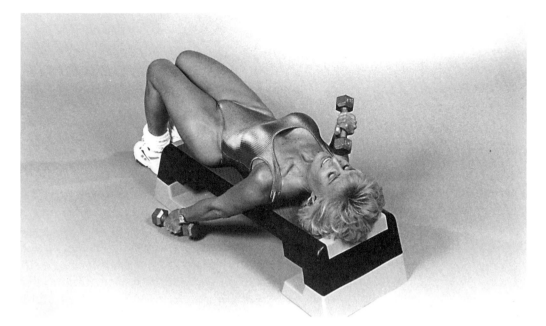

Position One

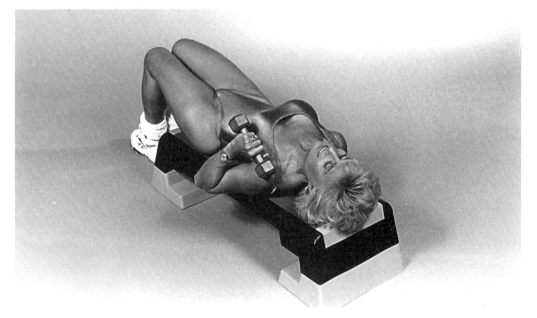

Position Two

Set 5: 12 reps lying simultaneous flat-bench curl, + 12 reps lying alternate flat-bench hammer curl, 1-pound dumbbells

Rest 15 seconds and move to the next exercise if you are doing the 30-minute workout. Stop here if you are doing the 15-minute workout.

THIGH ROUTINE
Superset: Squat (or Side Leg Lift) with Leg Extension

(Wonder Woman routine: add and speed-set leg curl. Dragon Lady routine, add and speed-superset leg curl with frog-leg front squat.)

I. Squat

This exercise develops, shapes, strengthens, and defines the front thigh (quadriceps) muscle, and helps to tighten and tone the buttocks (gluteus maximus).

Position: With a dumbbell held in each hand, stand with your feet about shoulder width apart and your toes pointed slightly outward. Let your arms hang down at your sides, holding the dumbbells with your palms facing your body. Keep your back straight and your eyes straight ahead.

Movement: Feeling the stretch in your front thigh muscles as you go, descend to an approximate 45 degree bend in your knees. Flexing your quadriceps as you go, return to start position. Willfully flex your quadriceps and repeat the movement until you have completed your set.

Without resting, proceed to the other exercise in this superset, the leg extension.

Beware: You may not be able to descend the full amount. Go only as far as possible. You may find that you rise on your toes as you descend. If so, you may place a board under your heels (optional). If you have problem knees, use the alternative, the side leg lift.

Machines, etc.: You may do this exercise with a barbell and plates and a squat rack, or on any squat machine.

SETS, REPETITIONS, WEIGHTS

Set 1: 12 reps squat + 12 reps leg extension, 1-pound dumbbells
Set 2: 10 reps squat + 10 reps leg extension, 2-pound dumbbells
Set 3: 8 reps squat + 8 reps leg extension, 3-pound dumbbells
Set 4: 10 reps squat + 10 reps leg extension, 2-pound dumbbells
Set 5: 12 reps squat + 12 reps leg extension, 1-pound dumbbells

Rest 15 seconds and move to the next exercise.

Start

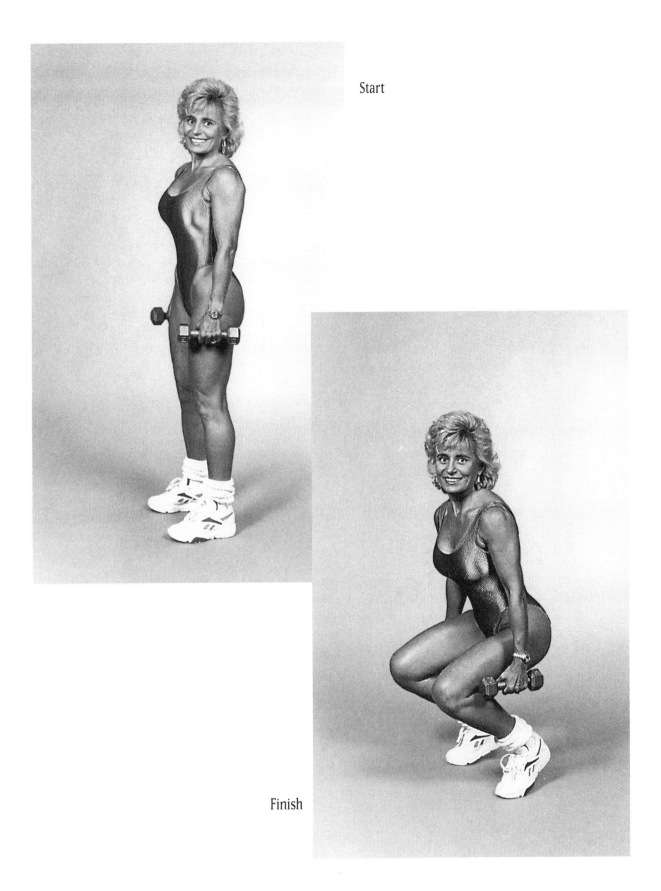

Finish

1a. Side Leg Lift

(Alternative squat for those with problem knees.)

This exercise tightens, tones, strengthens, and defines the inner thigh muscles, and helps to tighten and tone the entire quadriceps (thigh muscle).

Position: Lie on the floor on your side, supporting yourself with your elbow. Bend your nonworking leg at the knee and place the sole of that foot on the ground. Extend your working leg, and place a dumbbell in the middle of your working thigh area.

Movement: Keeping your working leg extended, and holding the weight on your thigh, flexing your working thigh, lift your working leg off the ground until you cannot go any higher. Keeping the pressure on your working inner thigh muscle, return to start position and repeat the movement until you have completed your set. Repeat the set for the other side of your body.

Without resting, proceed to the other exercise in this superset, the leg extension.

Beware: Flex your working inner thigh muscle as you raise and lower your leg.

Machines, etc.: You may perform this exercise on any inner thigh machine, at 20 pounds.

SETS, REPETITIONS, WEIGHTS

Set 1: 12 reps side leg lift + 12 reps leg extension, 1-pound dumbbells
Set 2: 10 reps side leg lift + 10 reps leg extension, 2-pound dumbbells
Set 3: 8 reps side leg lift + 8 reps leg extension, 3-pound dumbbells
Set 4: 10 reps side leg lift + 10 reps leg extension, 2-pound dumbbells
Set 5: 12 reps side leg lift + 12 reps leg extension, 1-pound dumbbells

Rest 15 seconds and move to the next exercise.

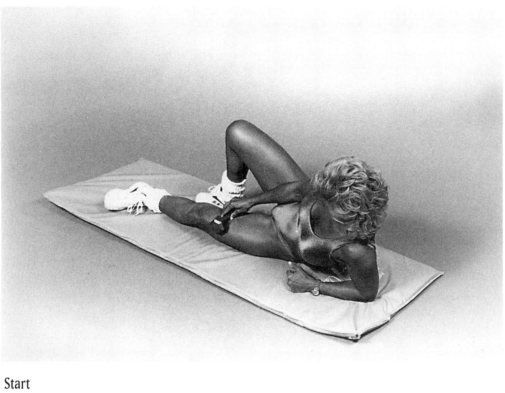

Start

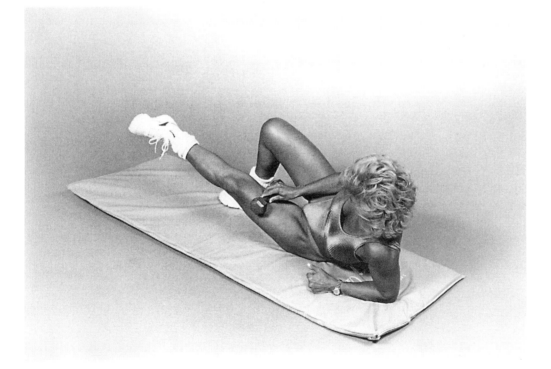

Finish

2. Leg Extension

This exercise develops, shapes, strengthens, and defines the entire front thigh (quadriceps) muscle.

Position: Sit at the edge of a flat exercise bench or chair with a dumbbell held between your ankles. Your knees should be bent and together, and in an approximate L position.

Movement: Holding the dumbbell securely between your ankles, and flexing your front thigh muscles as you go, extend your legs until they are straight out in front of you. Willfully flex your quadriceps muscles and return to start position. Feel the stretch in your quadriceps and repeat the movement until you have completed your set.

Without resting, perform your second through fifth sets of this exercise combination, the squat (or side leg lift) and the leg extension.

Beware: Don't try to do this exercise without sneakers. The weight will dig into your feet. You may use ankle weights instead of a dumbbell, but a dumbbell is better for flexing the thighs. If you can't do this exercise, double up on the side leg lift instead.

Machines, etc.: You may perform this exercise on any leg extension machine.

SETS, REPETITIONS, WEIGHTS

(same as page 148—repeated here for review):

Set 1: 12 reps squat + 12 reps leg extension, 1-pound dumbbells
Set 2: 10 reps squat + 10 reps leg extension, 2-pound dumbbells
Set 3: 8 reps squat + 8 reps leg extension, 3-pound dumbbells
Set 4: 10 reps squat + 10 reps leg extension, 2-pound dumbbells
Set 5: 12 reps squat + 12 reps leg extension, 1-pound dumbbells

Rest 15 seconds and move to the next exercise.

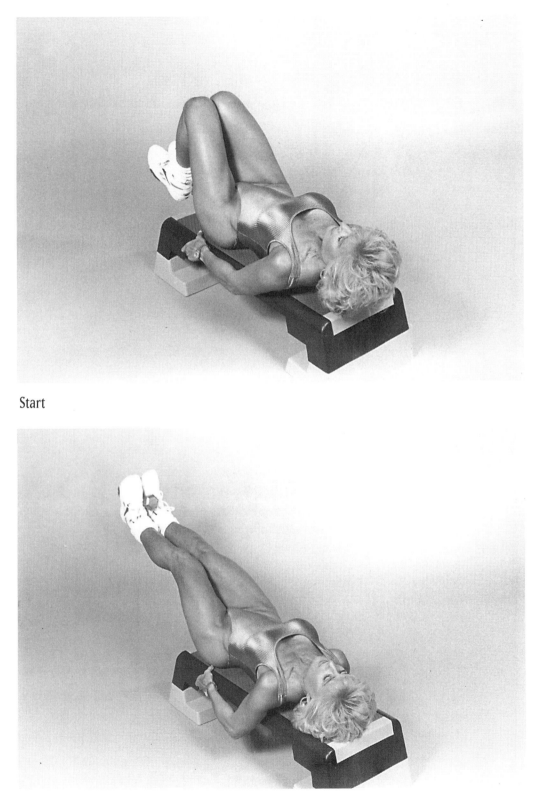

Start

Finish

3. Leg Curl

(For Wonder Woman routine: add and speed-set leg curl. For Dragon Lady routine: add and speed-superset leg curl with frog-leg front squat.)

This exercise tightens, tones, shapes, and defines the back thigh muscles (biceps femoris, or hamstrings).

Position: With a dumbbell placed between your feet, lie in a prone position on the floor or a flat exercise bench. Extend your legs straight out behind you and lean on your elbows for support.

Movement: Bending at the knees and flexing your hamstrings as you go, raise your lower legs until they are perpendicular to the floor. Keeping the pressure on your hamstrings, return to start position and repeat the movement until you have completed your set. If you are on the Wonder Woman routine, proceed to the next body part, the hips/buttocks. If you are on the Dragon Lady routine, you will speed-superset this exercise with the other exercise in this superset, the frog-leg front squat.

Beware: Don't swing the dumbbells up and down. If you squeeze your ankles together, you will be better able to keep the pressure on your back thigh muscles.

Machines, etc.: You may perform this exercise on any leg-curl machine.

SETS, REPETITIONS, WEIGHTS

(Wonder Woman routine):

Set 1: 12 reps leg curl, 1-pound dumbbells
Set 2: 10 reps leg curl, 2-pound dumbbells
Set 3: 8 reps leg curl, 3-pound dumbbells
Set 4: 10 reps leg curl, 2-pound dumbbells
Set 5: 12 reps leg curl, 1-pound dumbbells

Rest 15 seconds and move to the next exercise.

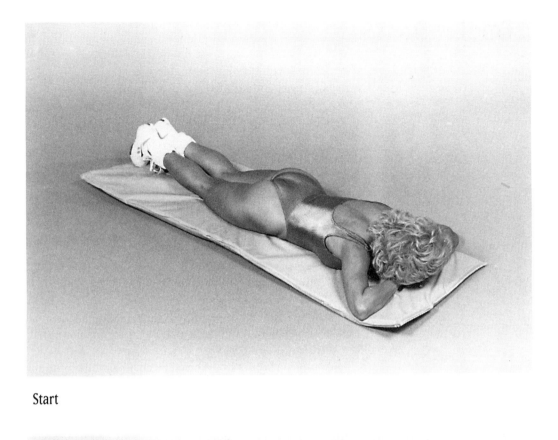

Start

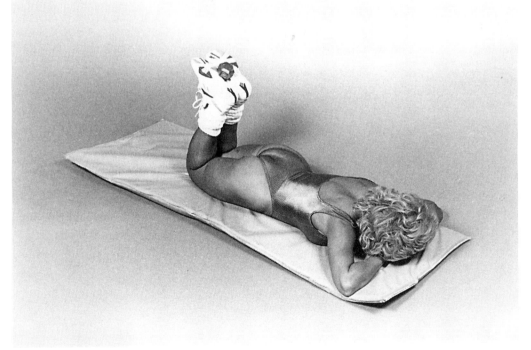

Finish

4. Frog-Leg Front Squat

(For Dragon Lady routine: speed-superset this exercise with leg curl.)

This exercise develops, shapes, strengthens, and defines the front and inner thigh.

Position: Stand with your feet wide apart and your toes angled outward as far as possible. Hold a dumbbell in each hand and cross your arms in front of your chest. The ends of the dumbbells should be touching your shoulders. Look straight ahead and keep your back straight.

Movement: Feeling the stretch in your front and inner thigh as you go, descend to a knee bend of about 45 degrees. Without resting, and flexing your inner and front thighs as you go, rise to start position. Willfully flex your front and inner thighs and repeat the movement until you have completed your set.

Without resting, perform your second through fifth sets of this exercise combination—the leg curl and the frog-leg front squat. Rest 15 seconds and then proceed to the next body part, the hips/buttocks routine.

Beware: Your anatomy may require you to rise on your toes as you descend. If this bothers you, you may place a board under your heels. Don't drop down or spring back to start position.

Machines, etc.: You may perform this exercise using a barbell and squat rack.

SETS, REPETITIONS, WEIGHTS

(Dragon Lady routine):

Set 1: 12 reps leg curl + 12 reps frog-leg front squat, 1-pound dumbbells
Set 2: 10 reps leg curl + 10 reps frog-leg front squat, 2-pound dumbbells
Set 3: 8 reps leg curl + 8 reps frog-leg front squat, 3-pound dumbbells
Set 4: 10 reps leg curl + 10 reps frog-leg front squat, 2-pound dumbbells
Set 5: 12 reps leg curl + 12 reps frog-leg front squat, 1-pound dumbbells

Rest 15 seconds and move to the next exercise.

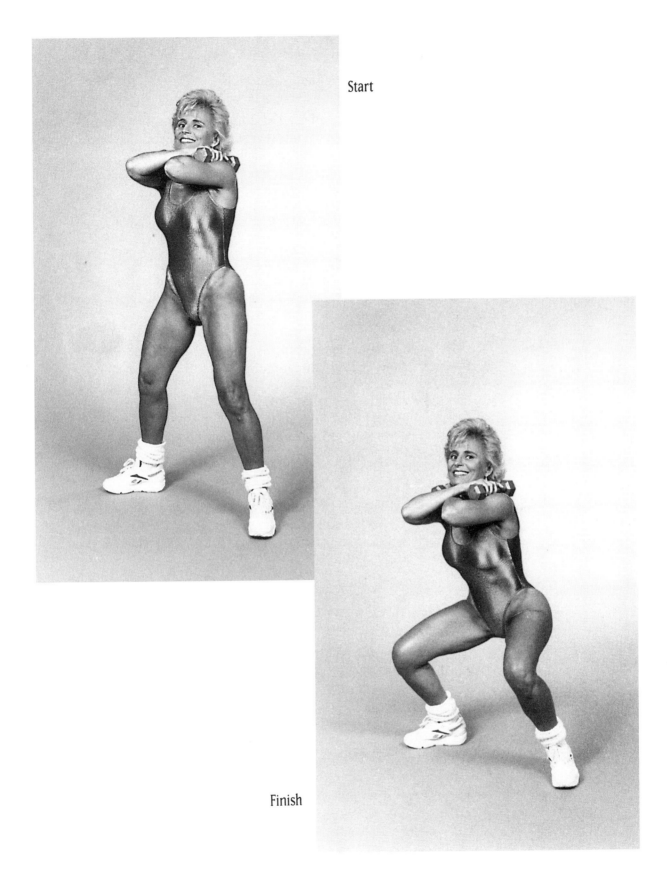

Start

Finish

HIPS/BUTTOCKS ROUTINE
Superset: Prone Floor Scissors with Prone Butt Lift

(Wonder Woman routine: add and speed-set horizontal scissors. Dragon Lady routine: add and speed-superset horizontal scissors with standing butt squeeze.)

I. Prone Floor Scissors

This exercise tightens, tones, shapes, and defines the entire hips/buttocks area, and strengthens the lower back.

Position:	Lie on the floor, on your stomach, and place your hands under your thighs. Raise your legs off the floor as high as possible. Your ankles should be about six inches apart.
Movement:	Scissor your legs together, crossing at the ankles, while at the same time flexing your hips/buttocks muscles as hard as possible. Continue this scissors-like movement until you have completed your set (double the reps, 15 for each side of the body, for a total of 30 reps). Without resting, proceed to the other exercise in this superset, the prone butt lift.
Beware:	Yes. This is hard on your lower back—but it strengthens the lower back. Take it slow and do only a few reps each time until you build up to the full amount. It's worth it. If you can't do this exercise, double up on the prone butt lift or the standing butt squeeze.
Machines, etc.:	You may substitute this exercise for any hips/buttocks machine exercise.

SETS AND REPETITIONS (NO WEIGHTS FOR THESE EXERCISES!)

Set 1: 15 reps prone floor scissors + 15 reps prone butt lift
Set 2: 15 reps prone floor scissors + 15 reps prone butt lift
Set 3: 15 reps prone floor scissors + 15 reps prone butt lift
Set 4: 15 reps prone floor scissors + 15 reps prone butt lift
Set 5: 15 reps prone floor scissors + 15 reps prone butt lift

Rest 15 seconds and move to the next exercise.

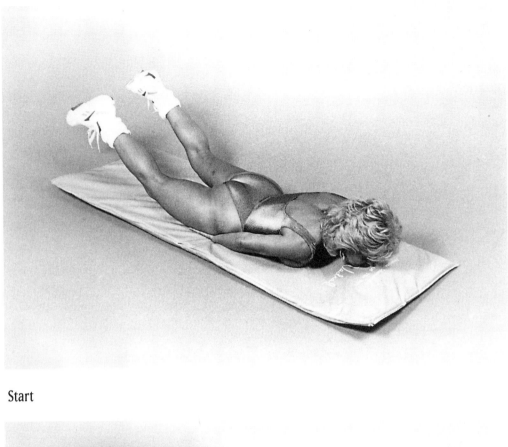

Start

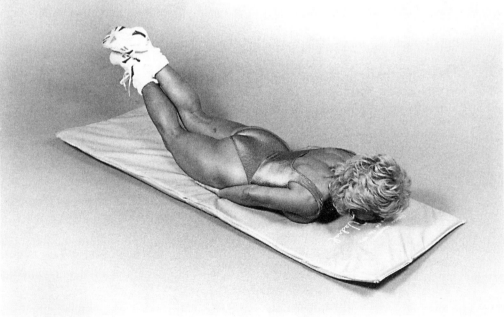

Finish

2. Prone Butt Lift

This exercise tightens, tones, shapes, and defines the entire hips/buttocks area, and helps to shape the back thigh muscle, and removes saddlebags from the side-thigh area.

Position: Lie on the floor on your stomach, leaning on your elbows for support. Extend your toes behind you, keeping your feet about a few inches apart.

Movement: Flexing your hips/buttocks muscles, and keeping your knees nearly locked, lift one leg until you cannot go any higher. Continuing to keep the pressure on your hips/buttocks area, return to start. Repeat the movement for the other leg. Repeat this alternate movement until you have completed your set.

Without resting, perform your second through fifth sets of this exercise combination—the prone floor scissors and the prone butt lift.

Beware: Don't tense your lower back. Relax as you work.

Machines, etc.: You may substitute this exercise for any exercise performed on a hips/buttocks machine.

SETS AND REPETITIONS (NO WEIGHTS FOR THESE EXERCISES!)

(same as page 158—repeated here for review):

Set 1: 15 reps prone floor scissors + 15 reps prone butt lift
Set 2: 15 reps prone floor scissors + 15 reps prone butt lift
Set 3: 15 reps prone floor scissors + 15 reps prone butt lift
Set 4: 15 reps prone floor scissors + 15 reps prone butt lift
Set 5: 15 reps prone floor scissors + 15 reps prone butt lift

Rest 15 seconds and move to the next exercise.

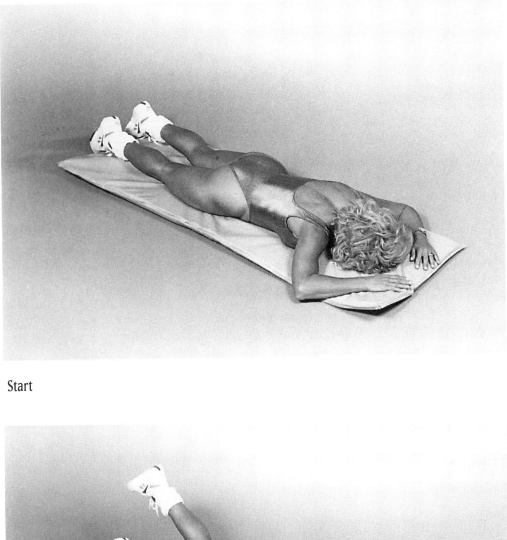

Start

Finish

3. Horizontal Scissors

(For Wonder Woman routine: add and speed-set horizontal scissors. For Dragon Lady routine: add and speed-superset horizontal scissors with standing butt squeeze.)

This exercise tightens, tones, shapes, and defines the entire hips/buttocks area, especially the outer area (saddlebags section).

Position: Sit at the edge of a flat exercise bench or a chair, and place your hands, palms facing down, under each buttock. Extend your legs straight out in front of you until your knees are locked. Point your toes forward. Your knees should be touching.

Movement: Flexing your hips/buttocks muscles as you go, scissor your legs apart until you cannot go any further. Keeping the tension on your hips/buttocks area, return to start position and repeat the movement until you have completed your set (you will scissor 15 times for each buttock, 30 in total for each set).

If you are on the Wonder Woman routine, proceed to the next body part, the abdominals. If you are on the Dragon Lady routine, you will speed-superset this exercise with the other exercise in this superset, the standing butt squeeze.

Beware: Be sure to keep maximum tension on your hips/buttocks area throughout the entire exercise, not letting up for a moment. Don't hold your breath. Breathe naturally.

Machines, etc.: You may substitute this exercise for any exercise performed on a hips/buttocks machine.

SETS AND REPETITIONS (NO WEIGHTS FOR THIS EXERCISE!)

(Wonder Woman routine):

Set 1: 15 reps horizontal scissors
Set 2: 15 reps horizontal scissors
Set 3: 15 reps horizontal scissors
Set 4: 15 reps horizontal scissors
Set 5: 15 reps horizontal scissors

Rest 15 seconds and move to the next exercise.

Start

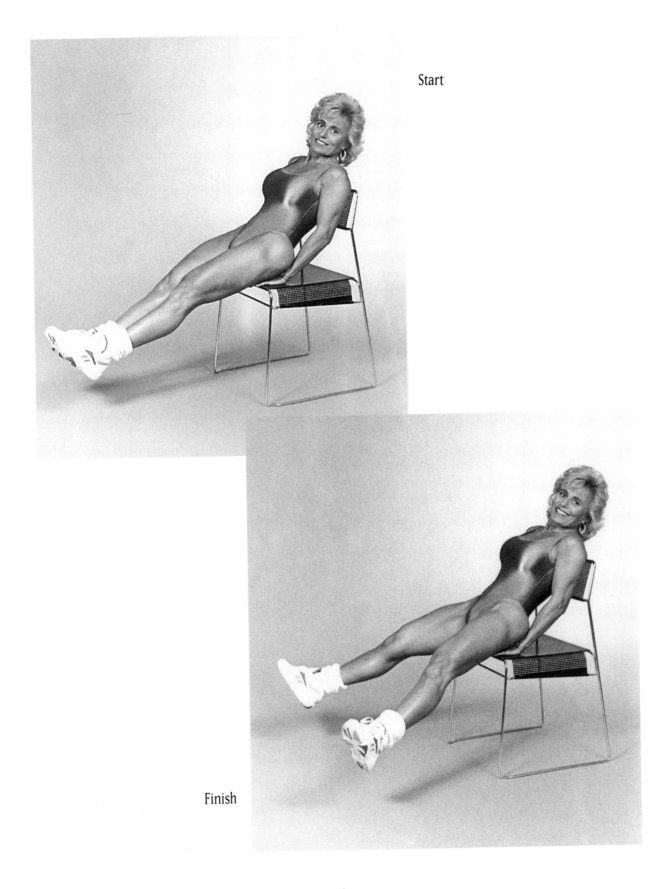

Finish

4. Standing Butt Squeeze

(For Dragon Lady routine: speed-superset this exercise with horizontal scissors). This exercise tightens, tones, shapes, and defines the entire hips/buttocks area.

Position: Stand with your feet a natural width apart and with your back erect. Hold a dumbbell in each hand, palms facing your body. Lower your body about four inches by bending at the knee.

Movement: Flexing your entire hips/buttocks area as you go, rise until your knees are locked, thrusting your hips slightly forward as you rise. Willfully flex your buttocks. Keeping the pressure on your buttocks, return to start position and repeat the movement until you have completed your set.

Without resting, perform your second through fifth sets of this exercise combination, the horizontal scissors and the standing butt squeeze. Rest 15 seconds and then proceed to the next body part, the abdominals.

Beware: The awkwardness of this exercise will quickly disappear once you get into the swing of it. (See video, *The Fat-Burning Workout: Volume II* for a demonstration of this exercise.)

Machines, etc.: You may substitute this exercise for any exercise done on a hips/buttocks machine.

SETS AND REPETITIONS (NO WEIGHTS FOR THESE EXERCISES!)

(Dragon Lady routine):

Set 1: 15 reps horizontal scissors + 15 reps standing butt squeeze
Set 2: 15 reps horizontal scissors + 15 reps standing butt squeeze
Set 3: 15 reps horizontal scissors + 15 reps standing butt squeeze
Set 4: 15 reps horizontal scissors + 15 reps standing butt squeeze
Set 5: 15 reps horizontal scissors + 15 reps standing butt squeeze

Rest 15 seconds and move to the next exercise.

Start

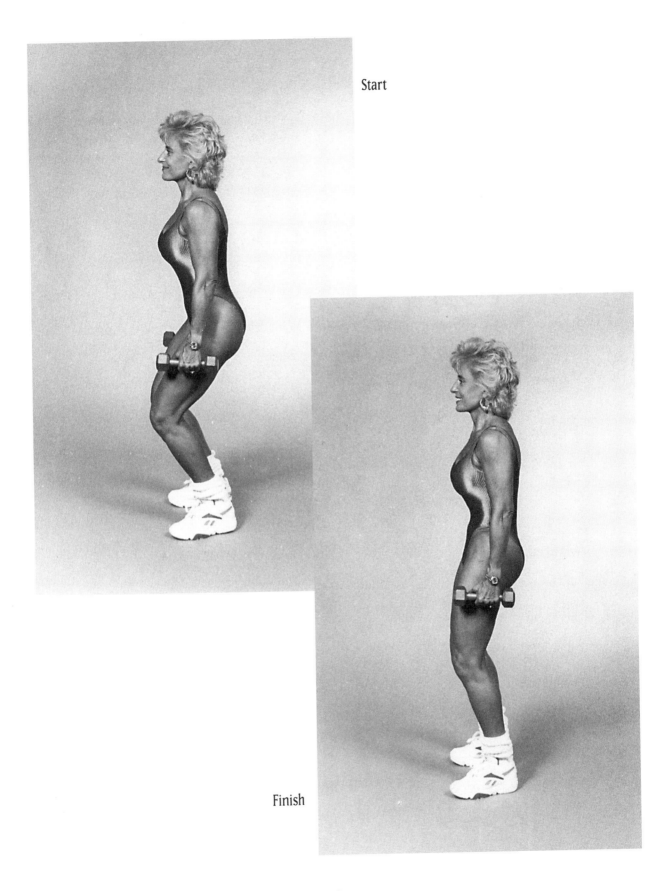

Finish

ABDOMINAL ROUTINE
Superset: Alternate Knee-in with Knee-Raised Crunch

(Wonder Woman routine: add and speed-set alternate twisting knee-in. Dragon Lady routine: add and speed-superset alternate twisting knee-in with side leg raise.)

I. Alternate Knee-in

This exercise develops, shapes, strengthens, and defines the lower and upper abdominal area.

Position: Lie on the floor with your legs extended straight out in front of you, but about three inches off the floor. Place the palms of your hands flat on the floor and under your back. Support yourself on your elbows.

Movement: Flexing your abdominal muscles as you go, bending at the knee, bring your left knee as close to your left shoulder as possible. At this point, begin to straighten your left leg, while at the same time beginning to bend your right knee, bringing it to your right shoulder. Continue this bicycle-like movement until you have completed your set (you will do 15 reps for each side, for a total of 30 reps per set).

Without resting, proceed to the other exercise in this superset, the knee-raised crunch.

Beware: Keep the pressure on your entire abdominal area throughout the exercise.

Machines, etc.: You may perform this exercise by supporting yourself on the standing abdominal step and alternately raising one knee at a time.

SETS, REPETITIONS, WEIGHTS

(Note: 1- to 5-pound weights are optional. If you choose to use a weight, place it on your stomach. Use the same weight for all sets.):

Set 1: 15 reps alternate knee-in + 15 reps knee-raised crunch
Set 2: 15 reps alternate knee-in + 15 reps knee-raised crunch
Set 3: 15 reps alternate knee-in + 15 reps knee-raised crunch
Set 4: 15 reps alternate knee-in + 15 reps knee-raised crunch
Set 5: 15 reps alternate knee-in + 15 reps knee-raised crunch

Rest 15 seconds and move to the next exercise.

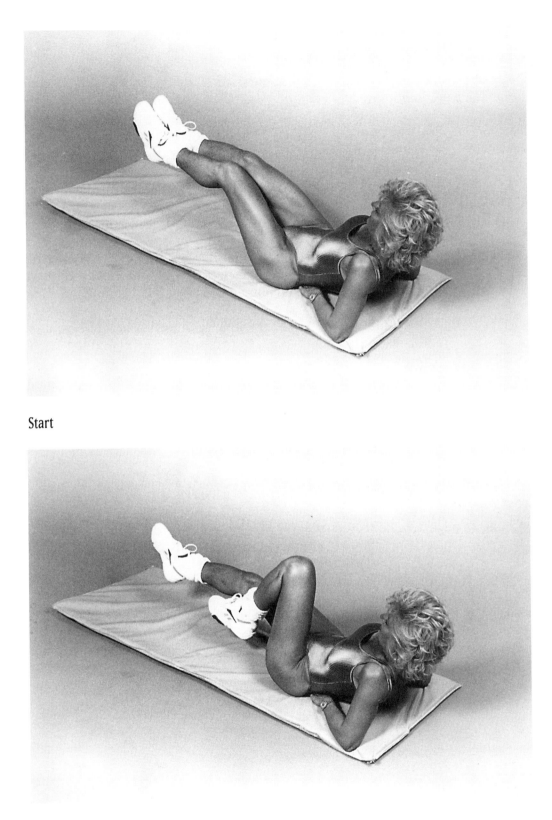

Start

Finish

2. Knee-Raised Crunch

This exercise develops, shapes, strengthens, and defines the entire upper abdominal area, and helps to strengthen the lower abdominal area.

Position: Lie flat on your back on the floor, and pull your knees up until your legs form an L. You may cross your feet at the ankles. Place your hands behind your head.

Movement: Flexing your entire abdominal area as you go, raise your shoulders off the floor in a curling movement until your shoulders are completely off the floor, all the time keeping your knees raised so that your legs are still in an approximate L shape. Keeping the pressure on your abdominal muscles, return to start and repeat the movement until you have completed your set.

    Without resting, perform your second through fifth sets of this exercise combination, the alternate knee-in and the knee-raised crunch.

Beware: This is exactly the same movement as the crunch, only it is done with the knees raised, so keep them raised and steady.

Machines, etc.: You may perform this exercise on any crunch machine.

SETS, REPETITIONS, WEIGHTS

(Same as page 166. Repeated here for review. Note: 1- to 5-pound weights are optional. If you choose to use a weight, place it on your stomach. Use the same weight for all sets):

Set 1: 15 reps alternate knee-in + 15 reps knee-raised crunch
Set 2: 15 reps alternate knee-in + 15 reps knee-raised crunch
Set 3: 15 reps alternate knee-in + 15 reps knee-raised crunch
Set 4: 15 reps alternate knee-in + 15 reps knee-raised crunch
Set 5: 15 reps alternate knee-in + 15 reps knee-raised crunch

Rest 15 seconds and move to the next exercise.

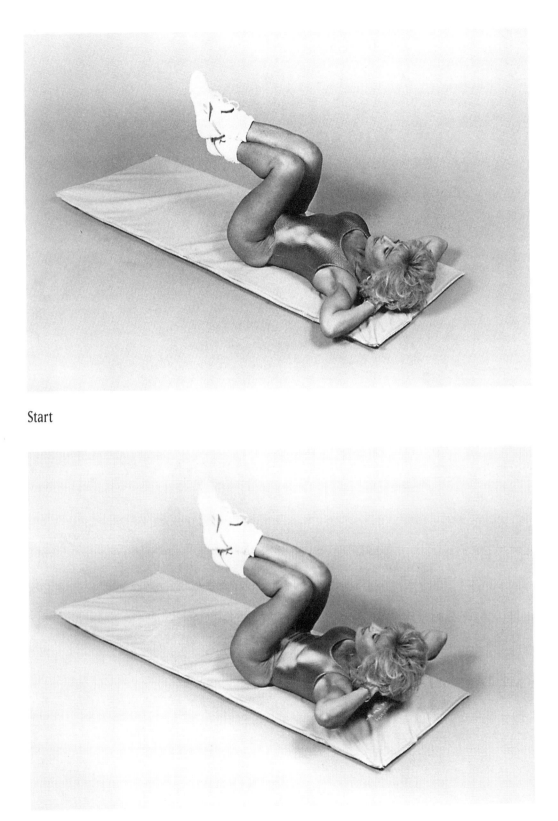

Start

Finish

169

3. Alternate Twisting Knee-in

(For Wonder Woman routine: add and speed-set alternate twisting knee-in. For Dragon Lady routine: add and speed-superset alternate twisting knee-in with side leg raise.)

This exercise develops, shapes, strengthens, and defines the lower abdominal and oblique muscles.

Position: Lie on your back on the floor or a bench, and place your hands behind your head. Raise your head a few inches, bend your knees, and place the soles of your feet flat on the floor.

Movement: Raise your left knee off the floor and simultaneously twist and try to touch it with your right elbow, all the time flexing your abdominal muscles. Return to start and repeat the movement for the other side of your body. Continue this alternate movement until you have completed your set (15 repetitions for each side, for a total of 30 repetitions per set).

If you are doing the Wonder Woman routine, complete your sets, rest 15 seconds and move on to your next body part, the back. If you are doing the Dragon Lady routine, you will speed-superset this exercise with the other exercise in this superset, the side leg raise.

Beware: Think of your legs as moving in a cycle-riding motion. Don't hold your breath. Breathe naturally.

Machines, etc.: You may perform this exercise on any crunch machine.

SETS, REPETITIONS, WEIGHTS

(Wonder Woman routine. Note: 1- to 5-pound weights are optional. If you choose to use a weight, place it on your stomach. Use the same weight for all sets):

Set 1: 15 reps alternate twisting knee-in
Set 2: 15 reps alternate twisting knee-in
Set 3: 15 reps alternate twisting knee-in
Set 4: 15 reps alternate twisting knee-in
Set 5: 15 reps alternate twisting knee-in

Rest 15 seconds and move to the next exercise.

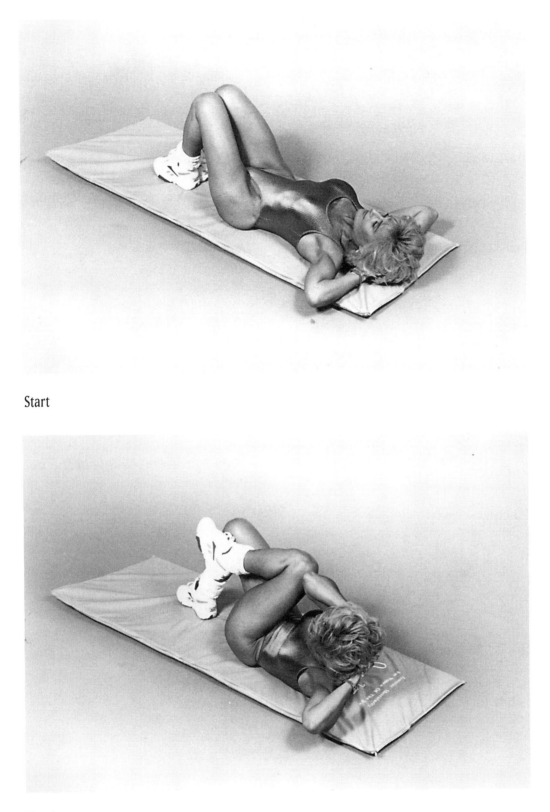

Start

Finish

4. Side Leg Raise

(For Dragon Lady routine: speed-superset this exercise with alternate twisting knee-in.)

This exercise develops, shapes, strengthens, and defines the oblique muscles, and helps to give the waist a smaller appearance.

Position: Lie on your side, supporting yourself with your elbow. Bend your lower leg to a comfortable position for support. Straighten your upper leg and point your toes forward and about an inch off the floor.

Movement: Keeping your upper leg as straight as possible, and flexing your side abdominal muscles (obliques) as you go, raise your upper leg until you cannot go any further. Keeping the pressure on your oblique muscles, return to start position and repeat the movement until you have completed your set of 15 repetitions. Repeat the set of 15 repetitions for the other side of your body.

Without resting, perform your second through fifth sets of this exercise combination, the alternate twisting knee-in and the side leg raise. Rest 15 seconds and then proceed to your next body part, the back.

Beware: Keep your hips glued to the ground during the entire exercise. They should not move at all. Concentrate on your side abdominal muscles, not your leg, as you work.

Machines, etc.: You may perform this exercise using a high-pulley device.

SETS AND REPETITIONS

(Dragon Lady routine. Note: do not use weights or ankle weights for this exercise.):

Set 1: 15 reps alternate twisting knee-in + 15 reps side leg raise
Set 2: 15 reps alternate twisting knee-in + 15 reps side leg raise
Set 3: 15 reps alternate twisting knee-in + 15 reps side leg raise
Set 4: 15 reps alternate twisting knee-in + 15 reps side leg raise
Set 5: 15 reps alternate twisting knee-in + 15 reps side leg raise

Rest 15 seconds and move to the next exercise.

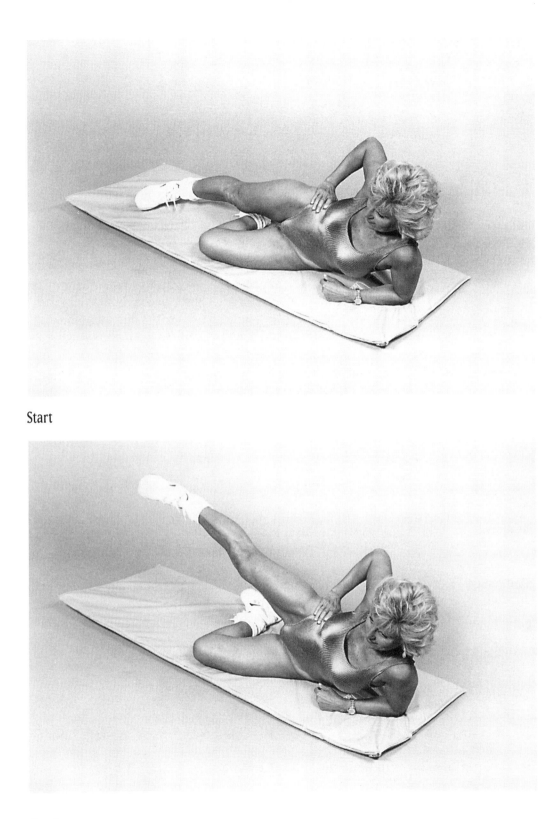

Start

Finish

BACK ROUTINE
Superset: Double-Arm Bent Row With Seated Back Lateral

(Wonder Woman routine: add and speed-set upright row. Dragon Lady routine: add and speed-superset upright row with double-arm reverse row.)

1. Double-Arm Bent Row

This exercise develops, shapes, strengthens, and defines the back muscles (latissimus dorsi) and helps to develop the biceps.

Position:	Stand with your feet shoulder width apart with a dumbbell held in each hand, palms facing your body. Bend over until your torso is parallel to the floor. Extend your arms straight down and hold the dumbbells in front of your knees.
Movement:	Flexing your back muscles as you go, raise the dumbbells up and out to about six inches away from the sides of your body, until you cannot go any higher. Willfully flex your back muscles and return to start position. Feel the stretch in your back muscles and repeat the movement until you have completed your set. Without resting, proceed to the other exercise in this superset, the seated back lateral.
Beware:	Don't rise to a near-standing position. Keep your back nearly parallel to the floor throughout the exercise.
Machines, etc.:	You may perform this exercise with a barbell or substitute it for the lat pulldown to the front or back, done on any lat-pulldown machine.

SETS, REPETITIONS, WEIGHTS

Set 1: 12 reps double-arm bent row + 12 reps seated back lateral, 1-pound dumbbells

Set 2: 10 reps double-arm bent row + 10 reps seated back lateral, 2-pound dumbbells

Set 3: 8 reps double-arm bent row + 8 reps seated back lateral, 3-pound dumbbells

Set 4: 10 reps double-arm bent row + 10 reps seated back lateral, 2-pound dumbbells

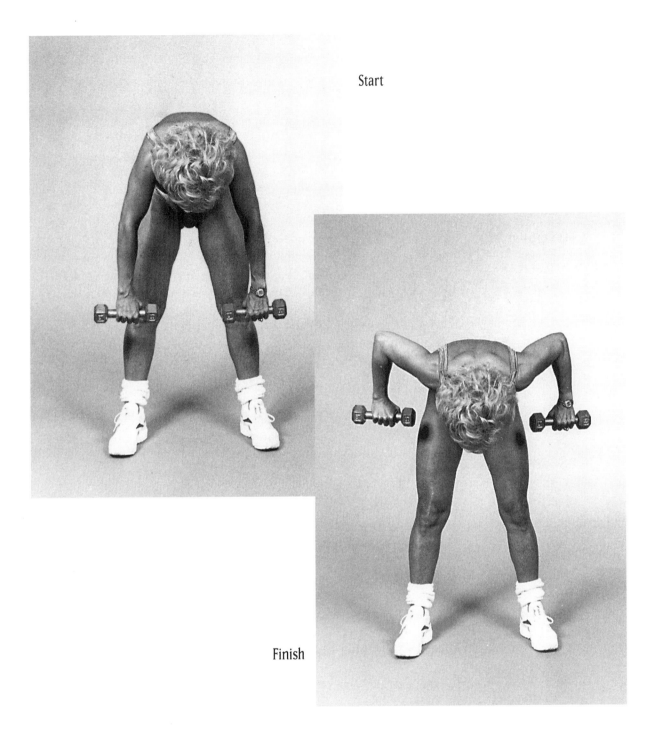

Start

Finish

Set 5: 12 reps double-arm bent row + 12 reps seated back lateral, 1-pound dumbbells

Rest 15 seconds and move to the next exercise.

2. Seated Back Lateral

This exercise develops, shapes, strengthens, and defines the upper back and trapezius muscles.

Position: Holding a dumbbell in each hand, sit at the edge of a flat exercise bench or step and lean forward until your upper body is nearly parallel to the floor. Palms facing to the rear, hold the dumbbells behind your ankles, letting the ends of the dumbbells touch.

Movement: Flexing your upper back muscles as you go, and keeping the dumbbells close to your body, raise the dumbbells up and back, rotating the dumbbells 90 degrees as you go, so that when you reach hip level, the dumbbells are angled to the front, and your palms are facing front. Willfully flex your upper back muscles by making believe you're trying to squeeze a pencil in the middle of your back. Return to start position and feel the stretch in your upper back. Repeat the movement until you have completed your set.

Without resting, perform your second through fifth sets of this exercise combination—the double-arm bent row and the seated back lateral.

Beware: Keep your arms close to your sides throughout the exercise.

Machines, etc.: You can substitute a T-bar rowing machine for this exercise.

SETS, REPETITIONS, WEIGHTS

(same as pages 174–175—repeated here for review):

Set 1: 12 reps double-arm bent row + 12 reps seated back lateral, 1-pound dumbbells

Set 2: 10 reps double-arm bent row + 10 reps seated back lateral, 2-pound dumbbells

Set 3: 8 reps double-arm bent row + 8 reps seated back lateral, 3-pound dumbbells

Set 4: 10 reps double-arm bent row + 10 reps seated back lateral, 2-pound dumbbells

Set 5: 12 reps double-arm bent row + 12 reps seated back lateral, 1-pound dumbbells

Rest 15 seconds and move to the next exercise.

Start

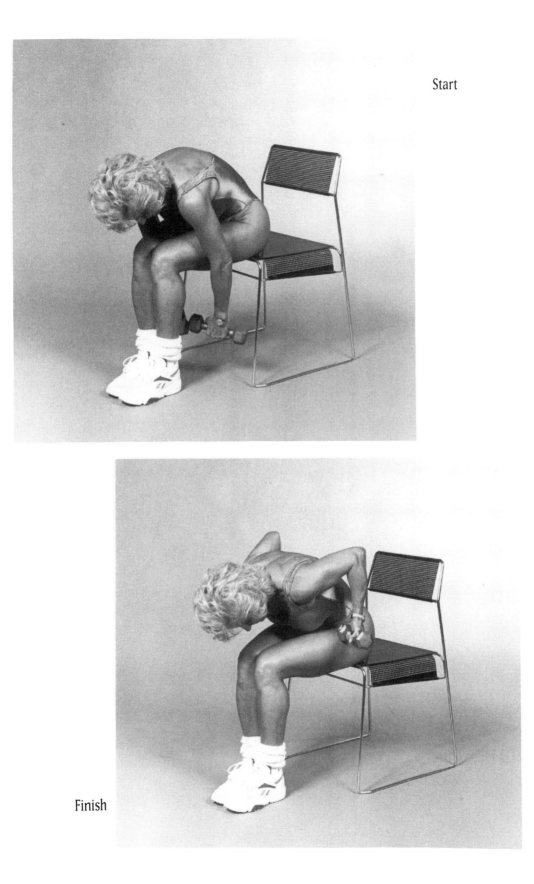

Finish

3. Upright Row

(For Wonder Woman routine: add and speed-set upright row. For Dragon Lady routine: add and speed-superset upright row with double-arm reverse row.)

This exercise develops, shapes, strengthens, and defines the entire trapezius muscle, and also strengthens and defines the front shoulder muscle.

Position: Stand with your feet a natural width apart, and hold a dumbbell with your hands on either end of the dumbbell, or with both hands in the center of the dumbbell, palms facing your body. Extend your arms fully downward and keep the dumbbell centered.

Movement: Flexing your trapezius muscle as you go, extending your elbows outward, and keeping the dumbbell close to your body, raise the dumbbell until it reaches chin height. Willfully flex your trapezius muscle and return to start position. Feel the stretch in your trapezius muscle and repeat the movement until you have completed your set.

   If you are on the Wonder Woman routine, proceed to the next body part, the calves. If you are on the Dragon Lady routine, you will speed-superset this exercise with the other exercise in this superset, the double-arm reverse row.

Beware: Don't let the dumbbell wander away from your body. Don't shorten the movement—go all the way up to your chin and let your arms extend fully down.

Machines, etc.: You may perform this exercise with a barbell, or by attaching a bar to any floor-pulley machine.

SETS, REPETITIONS, WEIGHTS

(Wonder Woman routine):

Set 1: 12 reps upright row, 1-pound dumbbells
Set 2: 10 reps upright row, 2-pound dumbbells
Set 3: 8 reps upright row, 3-pound dumbbells
Set 4: 10 reps upright row, 2-pound dumbbells
Set 5: 12 reps upright row, 1-pound dumbbells

Rest 15 seconds and move to the next exercise.

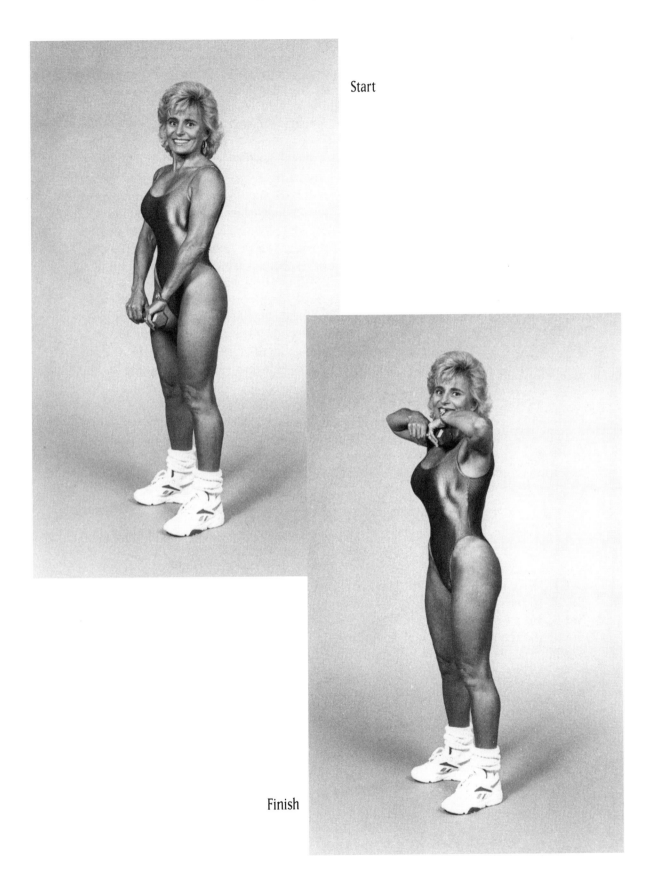

Start

Finish

4. Double-Arm Reverse Row

(For Dragon Lady routine: speed-superset this exercise with upright row.)

This exercise develops, shapes, strengthens, and defines the latissimus dorsi, the trapezius, the rear deltoid, and the forearm.

Position: Stand with your feet shoulder width apart, with a dumbbell held in each hand, palms away from your body. Bend over until your torso is parallel to the floor. Extend your arms straight down and let them touch the upper-thigh-knee area.

Movement: Flexing your back muscles as you go, raise the dumbbells up and to the side of your body (about six inches out at the highest point—waist height). Willfully flex your back muscles and return to start position. Feel the stretch in your back muscles and repeat the movement until you have completed your set.

Without resting, perform your second through fifth sets of this exercise combination—the upright row and the double-arm reverse row. Rest 15 seconds and then proceed to the next body part, the calves.

Beware: Maintain the near-parallel-to-floor position of your torso. Don't gradually rise up. Don't hold your breath. Breathe naturally.

Machines, etc.: You may use a barbell for this exercise.

SETS, REPETITIONS, WEIGHTS

(Dragon Lady routine):

Set 1: 12 reps upright row + 12 reps double-arm reverse row, 1-pound dumbbells
Set 2: 10 reps upright row + 10 reps double-arm reverse row, 2-pound dumbbells
Set 3: 8 reps upright row + 8 reps double-arm reverse row, 3-pound dumbbells
Set 4: 10 reps upright row + 10 reps double-arm reverse row, 2-pound dumbbells
Set 5: 12 reps upright row + 12 reps double-arm reverse row, 1-pound dumbbells

Rest 15 seconds and move to the next exercise.

Start

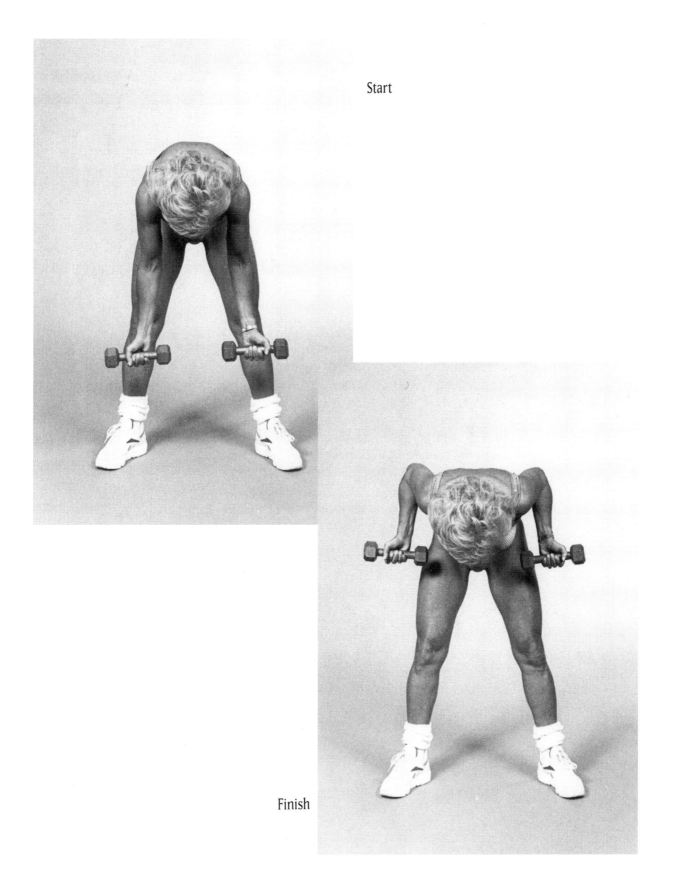

Finish

CALVES ROUTINE
Superset: Seated Straight-Toe Calf Raise with Seated Angled-Out-Toe Calf Raise

(Wonder Woman routine: add and speed-set standing straight-toe calf raise. Dragon Lady routine: add and speed-superset standing straight-toe calf raise with standing angled-in-toe calf raise.)

I. Seated Straight-Toe Calf Raise

This exercise develops, shapes, strengthens, and defines the entire calf muscle (gastrocnemius).

Position: Sit on a flat exercise bench or a chair with a set of dumbbells held on top of your knees. Plant your heels on the ground.

Movement: Keeping your toes pointed straight ahead and flexing your calf muscles as you go, raise your heels until you cannot go any further. Willfully flex your calf muscles and return to start position. Feel the stretch in your calf muscles and repeat the movement until you have completed your set.

Without resting, proceed to the other exercise in this superset, the seated angled-out-toe calf raise.

Beware: You have the option of placing a thick book under the balls of your feet if you feel that you are not getting a full range of motion.

Machines, etc.: You may perform this exercise on any seated calf machine.

SETS, REPETITIONS, WEIGHTS

Set 1: 12 reps seated straight-toe calf raise + 12 reps seated angled-out-toe calf raise, 1-pound dumbbells
Set 2: 10 reps seated straight-toe calf raise + 10 reps seated angled-out-toe calf raise, 2-pound dumbbells
Set 3: 8 reps seated straight-toe calf raise + 8 reps seated angled-out-toe calf raise, 3-pound dumbbells
Set 4: 10 reps seated straight-toe calf raise + 10 reps seated angled-out-toe calf raise, 2-pound dumbbells
Set 5: 12 reps seated straight-toe calf raise + 12 reps seated angled-out-toe calf raise, 1-pound dumbbells

Rest 15 seconds and move to the next exercise.

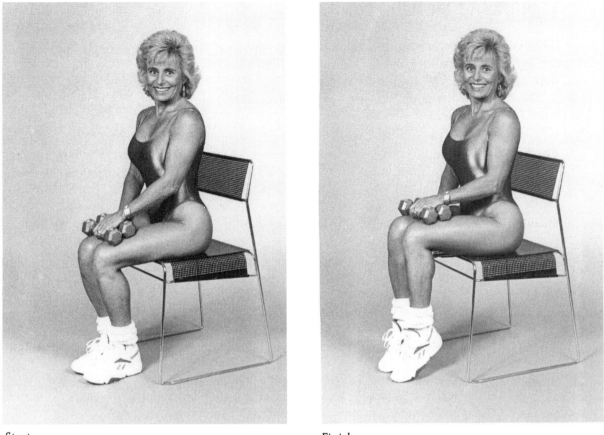

Start   Finish

2. Seated Angled-Out-Toe Calf Raise

This exercise develops, shapes, strengthens, and defines the entire calf (gastrocnemius) muscle, especially the inner area.

You will perform this exercise in exactly the same manner as the seated straight-toe calf raise, only instead of positioning your toes straight ahead, you will angle them out to the side as far as possible.

Without resting, you will perform your second through fifth sets of this superset, the seated straight-toe calf raise and the seated angled-out-toe calf raise.

SETS, REPETITIONS, WEIGHTS

(Same as page 182.)

Rest 15 seconds and move to the next exercise if you are doing the Wonder Woman or Dragon Lady routine. Otherwise stop here: Congratulations. You have completed your total-body workout.

3. Standing Straight-Toe Calf Raise

(For Wonder Woman routine: add and speed-set standing straight-toe calf raise. For Dragon Lady routine: add and speed-superset standing straight-toe calf raise with standing angled-in-toe calf raise.)

This exercise develops, shapes, strengthens, and defines the entire gastrocnemius (calf) muscle.

Position: Stand with your feet a natural width apart, your toes flat on the floor, and hold a dumbbell in each hand, palms facing inward.

Movement: Flexing your calf muscles as you go, raise yourself as high as possible. When you reach the highest point, willfully flex your calf muscles and return to start position. Feel the stretch in your calf muscles and repeat the movement until you have completed your set. If you are on the Wonder Woman routine, stop here. If you are on the Dragon Lady routine, you will speed-superset this exercise with the other exercise in this superset, the standing angled-in-toe calf raise.

Beware: You have the option of using a thick book under the balls of your feet if you feel that you are not getting a full range of motion. You will probably have to hold on to something in order to keep your balance—and in this case, you will not be able to hold the dumbbells. Don't worry. Your calves will still get a good workout—after all, they are supporting the weight of your entire body.

Machines, etc.:   You may perform this exercise on any standing calf machine.

SETS, REPETITIONS, WEIGHTS

(Wonder Woman routine):

Set 1: 12 reps standing straight-toe calf raise, 1-pound dumbbells
Set 2: 10 reps standing straight-toe calf raise, 2-pound dumbbells
Set 3: 8 reps standing straight-toe calf raise, 3-pound dumbbells
Set 4: 10 reps standing straight-toe calf raise, 2-pound dumbbells
Set 5: 12 reps standing straight-toe calf raise, 1-pound dumbbells

Rest 15 seconds and move to the next exercise if you are doing the Dragon Lady routine. Otherwise stop here: Congratulations. You have completed your total-body workout.

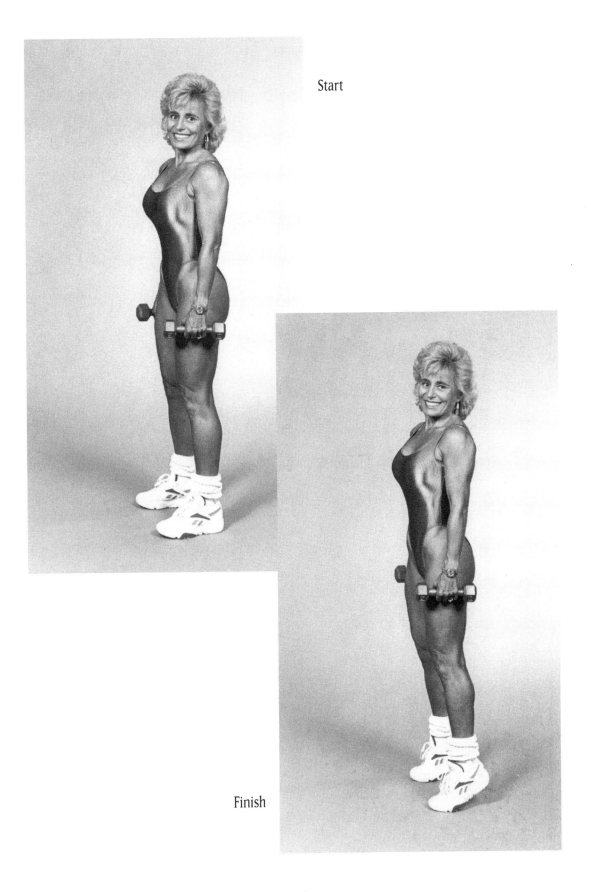

Start

Finish

4. Standing Angled-In-Toe Calf Raise

(For Dragon Lady Routine: speed-superset (this exercise) with standing straight-toe calf raise.)

This exercise develops, shapes, strengthens, and defines the entire calf muscle, especially the outer calf area.

You will perform this exercise in exactly the same manner as the standing straight-toe calf raise (see page 185), only instead of positioning your toes straight ahead, you will angle them in.

Without resting, you will perform your second through fifth sets of this superset, the standing straight-toe calf raise and the standing angled-in-toe calf raise.

SETS, REPETITIONS, WEIGHTS

(Dragon Lady routine):

Set 1: 12 reps standing straight-toe calf raise + 12 reps standing angled-in-toe calf raise, 1-pound dumbbells

Set 2: 10 reps standing straight-toe calf raise + 10 reps standing angled-in-toe calf raise, 2-pound dumbbells

Set 3: 8 reps standing straight-toe calf raise + 8 reps standing angled-in-toe calf raise, 3-pound dumbbells

Set 4: 10 reps standing straight-toe calf raise + 10 reps standing angled-in-toe calf raise, 2-pound dumbbells

Set 5: 12 reps standing straight-toe calf raise + 12 reps standing angled-in-toe calf raise, 1-pound dumbbells

Congratulations. You have completed your total-body workout.

REVIEW OF EXERCISES FOUND IN THIS CHAPTER

1. Chest

Flat flye
Flat press
Incline flye (W)
Incline press (D)

2. Triceps

Seated overhead press
Close bench press
Simultaneous kickback (W)
Lying extension (D)

3. Shoulders

Reverse overhead lateral
Bent lateral
Side lateral (W)
Alternate shoulder press (D)

4. Biceps

Simultaneous standing curl
Alternate reverse curl
Lying simultaneous flat-bench curl (W)
Lying alternate flat-bench hammer curl
(D)

5. Thighs

Squat (or side leg lift)
Leg extension
Leg curl (W)
Frog-leg front squat (D)

6. Hips/Buttocks

Prone floor scissors
Prone butt lift
Horizontal scissors (W)
Standing butt squeeze (D)

7. Abdominals

Alternate knee-in
Knee-raised crunch
Alternate twisting knee-in (W)
Side leg raise (D)

8. Back

Double-arm bent row
Seated back lateral
Upright row (W)
Double-arm reverse row (D)

9. Calves

Seated straight-toe calf raise
Seated angled-out-toe calf raise
Standing straight-toe calf raise (W)
Standing angled-in-toe calf raise
(D)

Fifteen-Minute Workout:	Thirty-Minute Workout:
Day 1: Do muscle groups 1–4 Day 2: Do muscle groups 5–9	Day 1: Do muscle groups 1–9 Day 2: Rest or do any aerobic activity

THE DEFINITION WORKOUT
TEAR-OUT WALL CHART

Once you learn the Definition workout you can use the convenient tear-out wall chart on the following pages. If you paste the six pages together you will have an overview of the entire workout in the order in which it is done.

9

THE DEFINITION DIET

Diet. The word has been abused and misused so much that we hardly remember its actual meaning. When we think of diet, we think of punishment, starvation, deprivation. But in reality, the word "diet" means: "food and drink regularly consumed." It's that simple. No big threat. So when I speak of diet, I'm not asking you to stop eating, or to suffer or deprive yourself. All I'm asking is that you change the food and drink you regularly consume from nonnutritious high-fat foods to highly nutritious low-fat foods.

I'm asking you to improve your regular way of eating, so that once you are in shape, you can occasionally eat whatever you please without guilt, or the fear that you will lose everything you worked for. In fact, I'm going to help you become so *comfortable with food* that food is *no longer a threat* to you. You'll make friends with food to the point where you feel once and for all in control in that area.

No one knows better than I do what it feels like to fear food and to feel that you can't control its effect on your body. First I feared it because I was underweight—and was forced to eat it—and no matter how much I ate, it didn't make me gain the weight I needed to gain. Then once I hit adolescence, and my female hormones kicked in, I began gaining. But when I got married, I continued to gain—at the rate of ten pounds a year, until I was fat.

I felt so out of control in the area of food that I eventually felt guilty anytime I put food in my mouth. "Something is wrong," I thought. "We have to eat in order to live. I shouldn't have to feel this way." Then I met bodybuilders, and I learned that you can eat plenty and *not only not get fat*, but *lose fat.* Soon food began to lose its mystery. I learned the rules. I knew exactly how to eat to lose fat, and I even learned how to indulge if I didn't mind gaining a few pounds of fat—because I knew exactly how to get rid of those pounds, calmly. I learned that gaining and losing fat is a science—nothing to fear.

NEVER GO HUNGRY—LEARN NEW EATING HABITS

The best part of nutritional eating is, you will never go hungry. You'll never have a moment when you will not be allowed to put food in your mouth if your stomach is growling—in other words, you will never have used up your food allotment for the day, because there are a number of foods you can eat anytime, anywhere, and as much of as you wish!

The fact is, you won't be giving up eating—not at all. You'll be learning new eating habits. But before you become comfortable with a new way of eating, you'll have to go through a time of transition—a time when you are teaching your body to recover from the bombardment of "sludge" that you have been feeding it, and to become accustomed to healthful eating. Once you do this (it will take three to six weeks), your body will actually cry out to you in protest when you try to stuff down an excess of fatty foods. In fact, your body will become addicted in reverse—instead of being addicted to fatty, sugary foods, it will become addicted to delicious, nutritious, low-fat foods of every kind. You'll see. It will happen—if you just cooperate and let it happen.

In this chapter you'll find the basic facts you need to know about good eating: calories and what makes us fat; the food value of fats, protein, and carbohydrates; and the place of fiber, calcium, and sodium, as well as vitamins, in the diet.

In addition, you'll find out how to diet for the long range if you want to stay lean and defined, and how to diet for a short time in order to look five to ten pounds thinner for a special occasion.

WHY WE BREAK OUT OF DIETS AND BINGE

We must feed our bodies in order to live. But there's more to it than that. We must feed our bodies a balanced diet in order to be able to forget about food and enjoy our lives; otherwise, we'll be constantly obsessing about food, and in addition, continually "breaking through" our best intentions and grabbing loads of foods we feel deprived of—in other words, going on binges.

A good example is what happens when you go on an extremely high-protein diet at the expense of nearly all carbohydrates. You can lose as much as ten pounds in the first week of such a diet, but it is not a fat loss—it's only a temporary water loss. You see, when you deplete your body of carbohydrates, your body flushes out water that has been held by carbohydrates in the blood and muscle tissue. Each gram of carbohydrate in the human body will hold four grams of water, so when you severely reduce your carbohydrates (to, say, only one half grapefruit a day and one cup of vegetables), your body releases its needed water (not the excess water that we retain when we overindulge in sodium—that will be discussed later).

But this is not a healthy situation. When carbohydrates are too low, your energy is low (your blood sugar level goes way down). In addition, you become irritable because the high-protein diet (say, double to triple the amount allowed in the regular diet found in this chapter) also contains high levels of phosphorus and low levels of calcium, upsetting the body's natural calcium-phosphorus balance. This causes what is called the "phosphorus jitters." You become nervous and irritable—ready to snap at anyone. So: what will happen once you are off guard? As a method of survival, if you should spy a bag of chocolate chip cookies, you can eat the whole bag in two minutes' time, even if you previously never had a particular liking for chocolate chip cookies, and when it is all over, wonder, "What in the world came over me? Why did I do that?" You did it because chocolate chip cookies have high levels of carbohydrates and simple processed ones at that—you get a quick fix of energy (and a load of fat calories with them).

People who go on unhealthy high-protein/low-carbohydrate diets for weeks at a time have no choice but to let their bodies go through the binge cycle—their only hope is to try to guide their bodies to eat the lower-fat, lower-sugar, complex carbohydrates instead of the quick-fix ones that the body pulls toward because of its "red alert" state.

The same red-alert state results from a severely low-calorie diet, such as a diet of 1,000 calories or under, or a liquid diet, where the body is deprived of its necessary chewing and the bulk that is needed to make the stomach feel full. In such cases, after a period of time, when your mind is not on guard, or at least when the diet is over, a "famine alarm" is set off and your body begins to binge on the highest-calorie, quickest-energy foods (fatty, sugary ones) it can find. That's why virtually all people who lose weight by starvation or liquid diets gain it all back within a year—and more in the bargain.

The secret for long-term weight loss is to follow a satisfying diet that does not put your body in a state of emergency, a diet that cooperates with your biological self. In other words, there's no sense in trying to follow a diet that in essence is like telling yourself to stop breathing. You can hold your breath for a minute, but unless you want to die, sooner or later you must breathe again, and when you do, like the binge-eating involuntary reaction, you will take in big gasps of air until you are feeling balanced again.

In this chapter, you'll find a *balanced* diet that fills your stomach with food anytime you are hungry. *The key word here is "balanced"—a diet that gives you just the right amount of the foods that make your body happy and allow it to forget about food and get on with the business of living.* In time, you will let go of your fear of food because finally you'll understand how food works. You will *feel* and indeed you will *be* in control of that area of your life, finally, and thankfully, forever.

Another reason people go off their diets is boredom. The human body craves variety. You can't eat the same foods day after day, week after week, month after month, and expect not to get bored. If you're bored with your diet, you will wrongly assume that you must go back to your old ways of high-fat eating, when the real problem will be lack of diversity in low-fat eating. That's why I want you to vary your foods, choosing from the lists of limited and unlimited complex carbohydrates, low-fat protein sources, and every conceivable fruit!

CALORIES—NOT THE BIG ENEMY

"How many calories?" Years ago, if you were trying to lose weight, that would be the big question before you could get too excited about a given food. People thought of calories as the enemy. Today we know better. We know that for the most part, fat, not calories, is the enemy, and the new question is: "How many fat grams?" You cannot, however, eat as many nonfat calories as you want if you want to lose weight (more about that later).

If calories are not the enemy, then what are they? Why do we need them to live? Calories are units of chemical energy released to your body when you eat and then digest food. Without the calories provided by food we would not have the energy we need to walk, stand, sit, or even breathe. In fact, without calories from food, we would die. So calories, in and of themselves, are not the enemy. Too many calories is the problem, but it gets more simple—because we can boil the problem of too many calories down to mainly one food source: fat!

HOW WE GET FAT

Since calories are fuel for your body, let's use the analogy of a car and the fuel used to run it: gasoline. If you try to put more gas in a gas tank than the tank can hold, the gas will spill out over the sides of your car, onto the ground. The extra gas would be wasted. A car has no special side storage tank to temporarily hold extra fuel if you overfill it. Not so with the body.

God, in His great concern for conservation of energy, provided us with an unfortunately foolproof system for storing excess calories, or fuel. If we consume more fuel than our bodies can use, instead of excreting it from a convenient valve, or even through normal processes of elimination such as sweating, urination, or bowel movement, our bodies store it for future use—and this storage takes place in the form of fat that is distributed all over the body, and in abundance in special storage areas, or, if you will, "tanks" (if the stomach, the hips, and the buttocks can be seen as tanks!).

I used to wonder why God didn't at least change the system once the days of the caveman were over. After all, storage of food for future famine is no longer necessary, at least in most countries. Why didn't He let our bodies evolve into a better system over time? Who knows? Perhaps God thinks we should be doing better things with our time than sitting down and watching television and eating all day and getting more and more bored and depressed. In fact, maybe He knew that if there were no consequences to overeating, many of us would spend our whole lives at the table!

HOW WE LOSE WEIGHT THE RIGHT WAY

You've heard this a thousand times. In order to lose one pound of fat, you must create a calorie deficit of about 3,500 calories. In other words, you need to take from the storage bin of fat 3,500 calories in order to get one pound of that flabby stuff off your body. You create this calorie deficit in three ways:

1. Expending more energy (by working out with weights, doing extra aerobics, performing sports, walking, shoveling snow, and so forth).
2. Adding lean muscle to your body—because muscle raises your metabolism and is active twenty-four hours a day (by doing the workout contained in this or any of my other books).
3. Consuming fewer calories by drastically reducing your fat intake!

We've already discussed the first two. The rest of this chapter will deal with number three. Let's talk about fat—the biggest calorie contributor—first.

Twenty to Twenty-five Grams of Fat Per Day: Why Is Reduction of Fat Intake the Best and Fastest Way to Lose Weight?

Simply put, fat has more than double the calories per gram than either protein or carbohydrate. For example, there are nine calories per gram of fat, while there are only four calories per gram of protein or carbohydrate. What does this mean? If you eat one gram of ice cream you've consumed nine calories, but if you consume one gram of pasta, you've only consumed four calories.

The next piece of bad news about fat is, it is so eager to store itself on your body (since it is already in its final form—fat) that it literally races through your digestive process using up almost no energy for the trip to your hips, buttocks, thighs, and stomach. Yes. Only 3 percent of the calories you consume in fat is used up in the digestion process of fat, whereas about 20 percent of the calories is used up in the process of digesting protein and carbohydrate.

Let's spell this out. If you consume 100 calories of pure fat, for example, if you dare to eat the skin of the chicken you just broiled, you've eaten 100 calories of fat and used up 3 percent in the digestive process, so ninety-seven of those calories are available for deposit on your hips. On the other hand, if you eat a baked potato of 100 calories, only eighty of those calories are available for hip deposit, because you used up 20 percent of them in the digestive process.

In addition to all of the above, eating that one teaspoon of ice cream, or that inch of chicken skin will not satisfy your food hunger—whereas pasta or a baked potato will!

In summary, fat is a very poor food bargain if your goal is to create the calorie deficit necessary to lose weight. I'm not saying that you can eat as much as you want of other foods and never get fat—I'm saying that if you lower your fat intake to twenty to twenty-five grams a day (how to do this will be discussed later in this chapter) you'll be able to eat a lot, a whole lot of carbohydrates and low-fat protein without getting fat. Of course if you eat ten pounds of pasta a day you'll gain weight. But who would want to do that? The truth is, after your first two pounds of pasta the pasta would get boring, and you'd be looking for other goodies, such as donuts and chocolate candy. So in reality, I can almost say to you, eat as much as you want of anything—as long as you keep your daily fat gram intake between twenty and twenty-five.

Well, No, Not Exactly—Why You Can't Quite Eat as Much as You Want as Long as It's Not Fat!

Almost. I said almost. Because some people find a way to overeat even though they are keeping their fat grams low. If you're more than thirty pounds overweight, you will still lose plenty of weight even overeating with nonfatty foods. It's when you get to that last thirty pounds that it gets tricky, because at this stage the body begins to fight you—it wants to keep extra fat in case of a future famine. You have to be very subtle and coax your body to let go of its storage supply.

The following sections will tell you all you need to know about the three basic food groups—fat, protein, and carbohydrate—and will tell you which foods you can eat in limitless amounts, and exactly how much of other foods you can eat and enjoy, and still lose weight and keep it off.

Fat: Some Is Needed to Live and Be Healthy

In order to function properly, the human body needs a certain amount of fat intake. It is fat that cushions the internal organs, and composes most of the cell membrane and sex hormones. In addition, if there is a fat deficit in the body, we cannot absorb and make use of calcium, or vitamins D, E, A, or K.

I can just see you now, foolishly worrying that you may not get enough fat in your diet. Put your fears aside. The average American consumes way too much fat in her diet because fat is everywhere (see discussion below). In fact, even those who think they eat a moderate amount of fat consume about 30 percent fat in their diet—better than the average American who consumes closer to 50 percent fat. The minimum healthy amount of fat consumption is exactly what I'm allowing you—12 percent to 14 percent. And in fact, you could go as low as 10 percent and still be in perfect fat-consumption health!

It is very hard to totally eliminate fat from your diet even if you tried. Fat is in so many seemingly nonfat foods, at least in traces. For example, even an apple has a gram of fat. The lowest of low-fat protein fish and chicken sources have about two grams of fat per ounce.

You Don't Have to Become a Mathematician and Figure Out the Percentage of Fat in Your Diet: Adding Up Your Daily Fat Grams Is Enough

I hate math, and I assume most people feel the same way. Yes. I had to pray my way through the math part of the Graduate Record Exams! God is good. I managed to get the minimum required to enter my Ph.D. program in English literature.

For this diet, all you have to do is count up your daily fat grams. If you can add, you can do it. When your daily fat gram intake hits twenty-five, you can have no more until the next day. It's that simple. And by doing this, you automatically keep your fat grams between 12 percent and 14 percent of your total caloric intake. (If I asked you to start figuring out percentages, it would involve you in division, or even worse, fractions—so I devised an easier method.)

But there's more to it than that. I don't want you to get bogged down in how much percentage of fat a given food has. For example, most food labels today have both fat gram counts and fat percentage counts. If you read a food label and discover that the food has only three grams of fat, but that it also has 40 percent fat, who cares. As long as you count the three grams into your allowed twenty-five, you're okay! See the math headache you avoided, and the enjoyment you can have in not caring what the percentage of fat is in a given food!

What About This Business of "Good Fat—Polyunsaturated" and "Bad Fat—Saturated"?

As far as getting fat goes, all fat is the same. "Good fat—that which does not clog the arteries," and "bad fat—that which does clog the arteries," both have the same amount of calories per gram—nine, and both use up only 3 percent in the digestive process, and both, in essence, go straight to your hips, butt, thighs, and stomach—as well as all over your body for storage quite readily.

If you follow the food guidelines in this chapter, you will not be in danger of overconsumption of even the "unhealthy" fats, because for the most part, the foods that contain them are forbidden until you reach your goal, and when you do, they are allowed only once a week—if you choose to indulge in them.

But for your information, let's talk about why saturated fats are considered more unhealthy than polyunsaturated fats. Saturated fats are found in animal products such as meat, full-fat milk, cheese, and butter—and in addition, a vegetable product, coconut oil. Except for coconut oil, they all become solid at room temperature, so you can see how they would easily clog arteries—and they do in fact tend to raise cholesterol levels.

Polyunsaturated fats come in liquid form and are derived from nuts, seeds, and vegetables. They do not solidify and do not raise cholesterol levels, but in fact make you just as fat as do unsaturated fats.

What Is Cholesterol Anyway?

Believe it or not, cholesterol is not a fat, but rather a fatlike substance that is found in nonfatty foods as well as fatty foods. For example, there is a good deal of cholesterol in shrimp, a low-fat seafood, as well as in red meat, a high-fat food.

Cholesterol is a natural component of our bodies. It helps to form adrenal and sex hormones as well as vitamin D and bile. Our cell membranes and nerve linings are composed of some cholesterol, and we have some cholesterol in our brain, liver, and blood.

You don't have to worry that you're not consuming enough cholesterol, because the body naturally produces its own. The big problem with cholesterol is over-, not underindulgence.

Cholesterol breaks down into two categories—"bad" cholesterol, which is labeled LDL, and "good" cholesterol, which is labeled HDL. The bad cholesterol, or LDL, can clog arteries by depositing itself on the arterial walls and forming plaque. When this happens, blood cannot flow freely to and from the heart, causing many problems, including a potential heart attack.

Good cholesterol, or HDL, in fact does the opposite of bad cholesterol. It removes bad cholesterol from the bloodstream and helps to transport it out of the cells and into the bile and intestines where it is eventually excreted out of the body.

In order to determine whether or not you have a cholesterol problem, you must find out the ratio of your good (HDL) cholesterol to your bad (LDL) cholesterol. A fractionated cholesterol test will take care of this. It will give you what is called an index. The lower your index, the lower your risk of heart attack. An index of four or lower is considered safe and healthy.

Indexes are determined in the following way. For example, if your total cholesterol level is 200, and your HDL is 50, your index is 4 (50 goes into 200 4 times), and you are in good shape. If, on the other hand, your total cholesterol is 200, but your HDL is 25, your index is 8 (25 goes into 200 8 times), and you are in trouble.

The point is, we must try to find ways to raise our HDL, or good cholesterol, while keeping our LDL or bad cholesterol low. HDL is raised by doing a workout such as this one, and exercising regularly in general. LDL is lowered by limiting your intake of saturated fats, alcohol, refined sugars, and caffeine, and by not smoking.

Forbidden Fatty Foods Until You Reach Your Goal

Stay away from all fried foods, and butter, margarine, and oil of *any* kind, lard, and chicken fat. Do not consume mayonnaise, or peanut butter. Forget about ice cream, sour cream, cream cheese, or milk that is over 1 percent fat. Run from beef, bacon, lamb, or veal. Forget about all nuts, seeds, or any kind of chips (potato, corn, etc.). Do not even dream of donuts, chocolate, or croissants. Put out of your mind cheese of any kind, and forsake olives and avocados.

Let's face it—you can't afford the fourteen grams of fat that is in one table-spoon of mayonnaise just because you like the way it tastes in your tuna salad. Learn to cook with spices and juices, or use the no-fat mayonnaise.

Sample List of Forbidden Fatty Foods—and Why

Food Product	Fat Grams

1 Ounce Cheese (one slice)

Cheddar	9.4
Colby	9.1
American	8.9
Roquefort	8.7
Monterey Jack	8.6
Munster	8.5
Edam	7.9
Swiss	7.8
Limburger	7.7
Provolone	7.6
Jarlsburg	6.9
Mozzarella	6.1

(Do you know how easy it is to stand at the open refrigerator and eat a few slices of cheese without even thinking about it?)

What about low-fat cheeses? I think they are still too high in fat. The lowest of low-fat cheeses have two grams of fat per slice (ounce) and the highest, nearly five grams per slice. To me that's too much fat for a small piece of cheese. But if you die for cheese, go ahead. Only be sure to count it in to your daily fat allotment.

What about No-Fat cheeses? Fine. To me they don't even taste like cheese, but you can have them. But be careful: see page 221—you can't eat unlimited amounts.

Fast-Food Hamburgers

Burger King Whopper Junior	20
Burger King Whopper	36
Burger King Whopper with Cheese	45
Burger King Double Whopper	52
Burger King Double Whopper with Cheese	62

(Better to indulge in a plain fat soft pretzel or a bagel—less than 2 grams of fat.)

Fast-Food Other Beef

Arby's club sandwich	30
Arby's super roast beef sandwich	28
McDonald's Sausage McMuffin with egg	27.4
Arby's turkey sandwich	24
Burger King ham-and-cheese sandwich	24
Hot dog	15

(Better to eat a gigantic slice of pizza—only 10 grams of fat—still not ideal but better than the above.)

Fast-Food Fried Chicken

4 ounces thigh	19
4 ounces drumstick	16
4 ounces breast	15

(Better to eat 4 ounces of any of the above broiled and without the skin—9, 8, and 5 grams of fat, in the order as listed above.)

Fast-Food Fish

Arthur Treacher's fried fish	19.7
Arthur Treacher's fish sandwich	19.2

(Better to carry a can of tuna in water—less than 1 gram of fat.)

Croissant Foods

Croissant	11
Burger King Croissan'wich with meat, egg, and cheese	24

(Better to eat a plain roll or two slices of bread—even with jelly on it—less than 1 gram of fat.)

Fast-Food Mexican Food

Corn dog	16
Jack in the Box super taco	17
Taco Bell burrito	20
4 ounces refried beans with sausage	32

(Better to eat 4 ounces of spicy beans—less than 1 gram of fat.)

Fast-Food Potato Dishes

Burger King french fries	22
Wendy's baked potato with cheese	24

(Better to eat Wendy's plain baked potato—less than 2 grams of fat—or any baked potato for that matter—less than 1 gram of fat.)

Fast-Food Dessert Products

Dairy Queen banana split	15
Large Dairy Queen ice cream dipped in chocolate	20

(Better to eat nonfat ice cream—no fat at all, or better, fresh blueberries or strawberries—no fat at all.)

To sum it all up, since you are allowed only twenty to twenty-five grams of fat per day, you will have to forgo the fatty foods until you reach your goal, when you can engage in them once a week if you choose to do so.

PROTEIN—THE BUILDING AND REPAIRING MATERIAL

By now you may be wondering, "Well, where will I get most of my twenty to twenty-five grams of fat? You'll get much of it in your protein—because most protein, even the leanest of sources, has some fat. But before we get into that, let's talk about what protein is, and why we need it in our diet.

Protein is the main building block of our bodies, and is essential to the natural repair system of the body. Skin, hair, nails, blood, internal organs, and most important, muscle, are made of protein. Protein also affects the production of the hormones that control metabolism, growth, and sexual development, and helps to regulate the acid-alkali balance of the blood and tissues, as well as the body's water balance.

Your ideal maximum protein consumption is about one half gram per day for each pound of body weight. (Bodybuilders often consume double that amount.) For example, if you weigh 130 pounds, sixty-five grams of protein is okay. There are about five grams per ounce of protein in poultry, and six grams per ounce in fish. So if you consume six ounces of chicken in one sitting, you will have consumed thirty grams of protein—one half of your ideal daily requirement. Since you are allowed two to three portions of protein per day, you can choose protein portions lower in protein grams for your other two allowances, have only one more protein portion for the day, or go over the one-half-the-body-weight amount (perfectly okay to do if your body seems to like it—muscles do like protein!).

You don't have to consume that much protein if your body or your doctor tells you no. In fact, the Pritikin Diet Center recommends about forty-four grams of protein per day for women as a minimum, and that's fine with me too, but in my experience, when you're building muscle, your body likes protein, so unless otherwise instructed, or unless your body tells you otherwise, try to keep your protein intake to about one half gram per pound of body weight.

The biggest problem with consuming too much protein is, it's easy to consume too much fat when you do, because that's where the fat is. Your low-fat sources of protein are found in white meat poultry, low-fat fish, beans, egg whites, and low-fat yogurt, milk, and cottage cheese. Details of daily allowed food portions are found at the end of the chapter.

CARBOHYDRATES—THE ENERGY FOOD

Carbohydrates are what give your brain and body the energy to function. They fall into two categories. The first is simple carbohydrates, or sugar, which itself divides into two categories: refined (sugars found in candy, cake, donuts, white flour, and so forth) and unrefined (sugars found in fruit). The second category is complex carbohydrates, which consist of vegetables, grains, rice, pasta, and fiber.

Simple carbohydrates provide immediate energy, whereas complex carbohydrates provide gradually released energy. First let's talk about the worst of the lot, simple refined sugars, then the next best of the lot, simple nonrefined sugars (fruits), and then the very best of the lot, complex carbohydrates—the all-day-long energy givers.

Sugar—Refined Simple Carbohydrates Are Not as Bad as Fat

Sugar is not as bad as fat, for the reasons discussed above, yet it is not the greatest thing if we want to lose weight. Why? If you consume it in excess, too much glucose is released to your bloodstream and this can cause your body to produce high levels of insulin, which hinders the enzyme responsible for pulling fat from the fat cells. So while sugar will not in and of itself make you as fat as fat (it has only four calories per gram, while fat has more than double that, nine calories per gram), it can slow down the fat-burning process of your body.

Sugar can also stimulate your appetite—the last thing you want to have happen. When there is an overproduction of insulin, as described above, the blood sugar goes directly to the liver, creating a blood sugar deficit in the circulatory system. This causes you to feel enervated, and this sensation of weakness signals you to eat!

Fruit Is Better Than Juice—But Why?

Both fruit and fruit juice are simple unrefined carbohydrates (sugars) but fruit is much better for you than juice. Although both fruit and juice are converted into glucose (potential energy) quickly, and both, if consumed on an empty stomach, can give you a quick energy burst and then a letdown (a drop in energy) fifteen minutes later, juice causes both a greater elevation and letdown because it is more concentrated than fruit—there is no food bulk to absorb the sudden dose of simple sugar. In addition, when you settle for the juice without the fruit, you give up the bulk that helps to fill your stomach and ease the feeling of hunger, in addition to the much-needed fiber provided by the bulk of fruit. Finally, you consume more calories with juice and still you don't feel satisfied.

In summary, the worst food bargain is the simple carbohydrates—processed sugars, for example, as found in candy. Then next worst is juice from fruit. And the best is fruit itself. You get a quick energy boost when eating any of these on an empty stomach—with an accompanying letdown. But with simple processed sugars, you are really being robbed, because in the (bad) bargain, you don't even get vitamins (at least with juice, although you get no bulk, you get vitamins), and with fruit, you get vitamins and bulk.

The point is, don't eat sugar, drink juice, or eat fruit on an empty stomach. Because the quick energy boost you get will not be worth the letdown you get fifteen minutes later when your blood sugar level drops, a letdown that gives you the urge to *eat* in order to pick up your energy. It's better to eat complex carbohydrates (and/or protein) first, and fruit after your stomach is at least partially full because this prevents a sudden drop in blood sugar and energy. Details on allowed daily fruit portions are discussed at the end of this chapter.

Complex Carbohydrates—The Best Deal in Town

Complex carbohydrates also fall into two categories: low-caloric density and high-caloric density. Caloric density is the number of calories per weight of a particular food. Since the human stomach can only hold up to two pounds of food, and most of us are not happy unless we eat until we are full, yet we want to keep our calories low so that we can lose weight, the foods that are low in caloric density are the best bargain because they fill your stomach without causing you to eat too many calories.

For example, vegetables (potatoes, sweet potatoes, yams, broccoli, cauliflower, etc.), pasta, rice, and hot cereals are low in caloric density (you don't have to eat a lot of calories of them to fill your stomach), while bread and cold cereals are high in caloric density (you have to eat a lot of calories of them to fill your stomach).

Let's take a closer look. If you wanted to put one pound of food in your stomach so that you could feel relatively full, and you wanted to do it with cold cereal, you would have to consume a pound, sixteen ounces, of cold cereal, and at about 100 calories per ounce, that would be 1,600 calories. On the other hand, if you were to try to do the same with potatoes, you would only have to eat four potatoes—about four ounces per potato—and you would only consume 400 calories.

What does this mean—that we should never eat bread or cold cereal? Of course not. It means that when you're really hungry and need that full feeling, don't try to fill up on these items. Use them for frills—and let the bulkier foods do the main job.

You will be allowed four to six portions of certain complex carbohydrates such as potatoes and pasta, and unlimited amounts of others such as broccoli and cauliflower. You can really enjoy your life now, because you know that no matter what, you never have to go hungry. For details on what is limited and what is unlimited, and how to incorporate them into your daily meal plan, see pages 229–231.

Why limit anything—as long as it's low-fat? Because if you want to lose weight, although high-fat foods are much worse for you than low-fat foods, if you eat more calories than you burn, you will not lose weight, and you could even gain weight. Not to worry—most people get bored with low-fat calories, but I don't want you to take that chance, so I give you a specific way to plan your daily meals at the end of this chapter.

One more point: As a general rule stick to whole grain or brown when choosing bread, pasta, or rice. The white varieties are processed and act as sugars—which can hinder your body's ability to burn fat.

WHAT ABOUT FAT-FREE OR SUGAR-FREE FOODS?

You have to really be careful about sugar-free foods, because they may be loaded with fat—and most of the calories (as discussed above) are in the fat, not the sugar. But what about fat-free foods? Here you have to watch out for an overabundance of sugar because sugar (as discussed above) can hinder your body's natural ability to burn fat.

But there's more to it than that. If you have to choose between low-fat and no-fat, of course choose no-fat. But don't get so carried away that you overindulge. For example, one of the substitutes for fat is Simplesse. It's made of protein from egg white in combination with no-fat milk products, and is now used in no-fat cheddar cheese. If you decided to go hog wild and, over the day, consume ten one-ounce slices, you would be consuming about 450 calories.

Take it a step further. Suppose you decided to eat a quart of no-fat ice cream during the course of a day, which has about 100 calories per four-ounce serving. You would add another 1,600 calories—a total of 2,050 calories. Now, if in addition, you consumed about 1,600 calories in other low-fat foods that are allowed in your meal plan, and you are in fact supposed to eat, you would have consumed 3,000 calories—too many calories for weight loss (even though I'm not going to ask you to count calories, when you are trying to lose weight, your calories should be at about 1,800 per day—never lower than 1,200, which is very low).

All of the above considered, if you do decide to indulge in no-fat or no-sugar foods, you'll have to count them into your limited complex carbohydrate category. See pages 229–231 for a guideline.

THIRTY GRAMS OF FIBER DAILY— FROM FRUITS AND COMPLEX CARBOHYDRATES

As it turns out, fiber is a very important diet component for achieving and maintaining good health, as well as losing weight and keeping it off! The good news is, if you follow the food guidelines above, you will automatically get the thirty grams of daily fiber needed for ideal health. In other words, you will get your fiber in your limited and unlimited complex carbohydrates, and in your fruits. After you read this section, compare the italicized words with the food lists below and you'll see exactly what I mean.

There are two types of fiber: first there is **soluble fiber**, which is found in *oat bran, psyllium, fresh fruits and vegetables, and legumes.* It can be digested by the body when consumed, and helps to lower blood sugar and cholesterol levels.

Insoluble fiber, which is found in *whole wheat, whole grains, celery, corn, corn bran, green beans, green leafy vegetables, potato skins, and brown rice,* cannot be digested by the body. Because of this, when you consume it, it does not register as calories—and in fact, the foods that contain them are automatically 15 percent lower in calories than they appear to be. Another great thing about insoluble fiber in the losing-weight department is, it acts as a fat vacuum, because when insoluble fiber exists in the body, some of the fat in your digestive system clings to the rough surface of the fiber, and as the fiber exits the body, it pulls the fat along with it.

Insoluble fiber also provides the stool with needed volume and helps to prevent constipation and eventual colon and rectal cancer.

WHAT ABOUT VITAMINS AND MINERALS?

If you follow the diet in this chapter, you will be getting all of your required vitamins and minerals from real food. But if you feel as if you want a safeguard, consult your doctor for a vitamin supplement. I don't take any vitamins or supplements. Food is all I need to stay healthy.

WHERE DOES SALT COME INTO THE PICTURE— AND DOES IT MAKE YOU FAT?

Salt, or sodium, is a mineral that is required by your body in order to regulate body fluids and maintain the acid-alkali balance of the blood. If you have too little sodium in your system, your muscles will cramp and even shrink—because it is sodium that is responsible for muscle contraction.

Sodium does not make you fat—but an excess of it causes you to retain excess water (it holds about fifty times its own weight in water) and temporarily causes your weight to go up—and in addition, to make you feel bloated. Perhaps this is why so many people have the misguided idea that in order to lose weight, they must keep their sodium level low.

The fact is, unless your doctor specifically recommends a low-sodium diet, you should keep your sodium intake at a normal level (1,500 to 2,500 milligrams per day). If you are trying to keep your fat intake low, you are already using quite a bit of discipline when it comes to eating. Why torture yourself with additional restrictions unless your doctor says you must do it for your health? For example, why not indulge in a few delicious long pretzels, not the low-sodium kind (about 400 milligrams of sodium for three pretzels weighing about ten grams each), and in fact if you're anything like me, maybe even eat ten of them at a sitting for a total sodium consumption of over 1,300 milligrams!

If you follow the eating guidelines in this chapter, you won't have to worry about getting your daily minimum of sodium. All foods have some sodium in them. For example, look how much sodium is found in seven ounces of the following nutritious foods.

7 Ounces of Food Item	Milligrams of Sodium
Cantaloupe	24
Carrots (fresh or frozen)	70
Carrots (canned)	640
Celery	50
Onions	20
Peas (fresh or frozen)	2
Peas (canned)	500
Potatoes	6
Chicken	100
Flounder	160
Canned tuna in water	600
Canned tuna in water rinsed thoroughly	200

The fact is, high-sodium foods always make you feel a bit bloated, but if you feel like indulging, as long as you stick to the low-fat healthier foods, your weight gain and bloat will be temporary. The big thing is, however, not to let that sensation of feeling fat fool you into thinking, "Oh well. I'm blowing up like a balloon. I might as well go to town and eat anything I want," and then start eating fatty foods. Instead, control yourself and realize that after about four days of moderate- to low-sodium eating, your bloat and water retention will be gone.

DO YOU REALLY HAVE TO DRINK WATER?

Well, you don't have to, but you should. I have the devil of a time drinking just plain old water. I do drink lots of liquids during the day, so my body does not scream at me, drink water. But liquids are not the same as plain old water. Plain water does your body the biggest favor—because it gives your internal organs a clean shower—instead of the usual fare of coffee, soda, and soup.

It is plain water that will flush out the excess sodium in your system, and in fact help you to not retain water! In fact, when you're trying to get rid of water bloat because of excessive indulgence in high-sodium foods, drink lots of water.

More than half of our body weight is water. We could live for a month without eating, but we could only survive a few days without water, because the human body loses three quarts of water per day through perspiration and excretion. Our body cannot store excess water the way it stores excess food fuel (it stores excess calories as fat).

Water is the basis of all body fluids, including digestive juices, blood, urine, lymph, and perspiration. It is the primary carrier of nutrients throughout the body, and is involved in nearly every body function, including absorption and digestion, excretion, circulation, lubrication, and regulation of body temperature. Water also helps the skin to appear moist and healthy.

How much water should we drink daily, in addition to any other liquid consumption for ideal health? Five eight-ounce glasses of water a day are perfect. If you have one glass of water when you awake, and one when you go to bed, plus one before each of your three major meals (it will also help you to feel full faster), you will cover the minimum five glasses right there.

CALCIUM AS AN INSURANCE POLICY

We've already discussed the bone-building power of this workout. But it's not enough to just work out. You must also feed your body the appropriate amount of calcium in order to insure that your bones do not thin and shorten as you age. Most doctors agree that 1,500 milligrams of calcium daily is a healthy minimum amount for women of every age, and especially for women over thirty. Here is a list of foods that contain calcium.

100 MILLIGRAMS OF CALCIUM

8 ounces skim milk
8 ounces low-fat yogurt
8 ounces low-fat cottage cheese
8 ounces cooked farina
8 ounces cooked Cream of Wheat
6 ounces cooked oatmeal
8 ounces navy beans
8 ounces soybeans

8 ounces broccoli
8 ounces collard greens
8 ounces mustard greens
8 ounces dandelion greens
8 ounces turnip greens
8 ounces kale
4 ounces shrimp
4 ounces scallops

There is calcium in many other foods as well. Get a copy of *The Nutrition Almanac* (see Bibliography) and become familiar with where to find calcium! If you are not sure that you're getting enough calcium in your diet, see your doctor about taking a supplement.

CAFFEINE, ALCOHOL, AND OTHER CONTROVERSIAL FOODS

Coffee's reputation varies from year to year. Depending upon the study, in moderation, it is good for your heart and increases energy, or it is bad for your heart and causes irregularities, fibrocystic breast tissue, stress, decreased blood flow to the brain, nausea, insomnia, fast pulse, increased need to urinate, raised cholesterol levels, and even decreased ability to absorb calcium!

I must confess that I enjoy my coffee—regular, perked coffee, and I guiltlessly drink about three cups a day. I have already proven that I am not addicted and incapable of giving up coffee by stopping coffee consumption for almost a year. I did have a headache for the first three days, but after that I was fine. Why did I resume coffee drinking? Simply put, I missed it. I just plain old missed it. Coffee in the morning is one of my motivations for getting out of bed. I hope I never have to give it up.

If you enjoy an occasional drink, fine—as long as you keep it down to one or two drinks a week at most. I don't recommend a drink a day because alcohol tends to lower your metabolism for an hour or two after you drink it—and it cuts your energy level.

If you're going to indulge, I say save it for the weekend, when you can have a drink or two on a Friday and/or Saturday evening, or some such thing. Yes. You can indulge in a drink or two even while you're on the strictest diet, but keep your drinks down to either white or red wine, champagne, or drinks mixed with juice or diet soda. Otherwise the calories add up quickly and you defeat your fat-loss plan.

YOUR DAILY MEAL PLANS AND HOW TO MAKE THEM UP WITH VARIETY

Here are your simple guidelines. Each day you are allowed the following—but you must in addition remember to count the fat grams and make sure that you don't go over twenty-five grams for the day. Note that I give you the fat grams when I list the specific foods. Also, for your information, remembering that it is a good idea to consume about half a gram per pound of your body weight in protein but not less than forty-five grams (bodybuilders consume even more than that), I remind you of how many grams of protein per ounce each food product has. First the portions, then the specific foods and their protein- and fat-gram content.

PROTEIN: 2-3 PORTIONS

One portion is:

4-6 ounces of poultry or fish, cooked
6 ounces of yogurt or cottage cheese
8 ounces of low-fat or skim milk
4 ounces of beans
4 ounces of tofu

LOW-FAT SOURCES OF PROTEIN

Poultry	Grams of Fat per 4 Ounces

All poultry has about 5 grams of protein per ounce

Turkey breast	2
Turkey drumstick	4
Turkey thigh	5
Chicken breast	5
Chicken drumstick	8
Chicken thigh	9

Fish	Grams of Fat per 6 Ounces

All fish has about 6 grams of protein per ounce

Haddock	0.03
Red snapper	0.7
Cod	0.9
Abalone	0.9
Sea bass	1.5
Sole	2.4
Flounder	2.4
Squid	2.7
Tuna in water	3.0
Pike	3.0
Halibut	3.6
Scallops	4.2
Brook trout	6.3

OTHER SOURCES OF PROTEIN

Food Product	Grams of Protein	Grams of Fat
4 ounces low-fat yogurt	6	1.75
4 ounces no-fat yogurt	6	0.0
8 ounces 1-percent-fat milk	8	2.6
8 ounces skim milk	8	0.4
4 ounces 1 percent low-fat cottage cheese	2	1.0
4 ounces full-fat cottage cheese	2	5.0 (No, no, no)
3 egg whites	10	0.0
½ cup beans	8	0.4
½ cup tofu	8	4.5

SIMPLE CARBOHYDRATES: 2–4 PORTIONS

1 portion is:

1 large apple
1 small banana
1 medium pear
1 large kiwi fruit
1 small mango
1 large nectarine
1 large orange
1 large peach
4 ounces no-fat ice cream
100 calories no-fat cake
100 calories fruit-based jam, jelly

4 apricots
20 grapes
3 kumquats
3 persimmons
2 plums
2 fresh prunes
2 tangerines
15 large cherries
100 calories hard candy

1 cup berries (any kind)
1 cup papaya
1½ cups strawberries
1½ cups watermelon
½ cantaloupe
½ grapefruit
¼ large pineapple
½ large plantain
¼ honeydew melon
1 tablespoon sugary jelly, jam

LIMITED COMPLEX CARBOHYDRATES: 4–6 PORTIONS

Breads, cereals, grains   Vegetables

One portion is:

½ bagel
2 slices bread
1 English muffin
8 low-fat crackers
4 rice cakes
1 pita bread
1 ounce cold cereal
1 ounce hot cereal
  (before cooking)
4 ounces pasta (before
  cooking)
⅔ cup rice, cooked

1 large baked potato
1 medium yam
1 medium sweet potato
1 cup corn
1 large corn on the cob
½ cup beans or lentils
  of any kind
1 cup peas of any kind
1 cup beets
1 ounce pretzels
100 calories no-sugar
  cake, etc.

100–120 calories *any*
  soup, preferably
  moderate-sodium,
  health-conscious
  brands

UNLIMITED COMPLEX CARBOHYDRATES: MINIMUM 3–5 CUPS, PREFERABLY MORE

Asparagus
Broccoli
Brussels sprouts
Cabbage
Cauliflower
Celery
Collard greens
Cucumber
Eggplant
Green or yellow beans

Kale
Lettuce
Mushrooms
Carrots
Peppers—red, green,
  yellow
Spinach
Sprouts
Summer squash
Tomatoes
Zucchini

Frozen mixed
  vegetables
*Any spices
*Plain or any flavor
  vinegar
*Lemon or lime juice
*Diet soda, club soda,
  seltzer
*Coffee, tea, any no-
  calorie beverage

Note: It is okay to count mixed vegetables as unlimited complex carbohydrates even though they may have some corn, beans, or other foods in them from the list of limited complex carbohydrates. For the most part, the frozen mixed vegetables will consist of unlimited complex carbohydrates, so don't worry. Enjoy. Also note that although the food items marked with an asterisk are not complex carbohydrates, they are allowed in unlimited portions, so I include them in this list.

Making Your Daily Meal Plans

Your first question is probably: "How do I know whether to eat the minimum or maximum portions allowed?" To answer your question, I will say that I always eat the maximum portion, and also a huge amount of the free, unlimited complex carbohydrates.

In the past, I have given you three to seven sample meal plans in a book. But my readers mistook those plans to mean that they had to keep repeating them, and keep eating those same old foods over and over again, or they asked me to make up more meal plans. Neither is a good idea. I want you to make up your own meal plans, based upon the food lists above. So now I'm going to give you a meal plan form, and you are going to learn to create your own daily meal plans. Here's how.

SAMPLE MEAL PLAN FORM A

Breakfast

1 portion protein
1 portion limited complex
  carbohydrates
1 fruit

Snack

1 fruit
1 cup unlimited complex
  carbohydrates

Lunch

1 portion protein
1 portion limited complex
  carbohydrates
1 fruit
1 cup unlimited complex
  carbohydrates

SAMPLE MEAL PLAN FORM B

Breakfast

2 portions limited complex
  carbohydrates

Snack

1 portion protein

Lunch

2 portions unlimited complex
  carbohydrates
1 fruit

Snack	**Snack**
1 portion limited complex carbohydrates	1 cup unlimited complex carbohydrates

Dinner	**Dinner**
1 portion limited complex carbohydrates 1 portion protein 2 cups unlimited complex carbohydrates 1 fruit	2 portions limited complex carbohydrates 1 portion protein 2 cups unlimited complex carbohydrates 2 fruits

Snack	**Snack**
1 portion limited complex carbohydrates 1 cup unlimited complex carbohydrates	1 portion protein 2 cups unlimited complex carbohydrates 1 fruit

Notice that you can move around your food allotment to any time of the day or night—and you can double up when you want to do so—except for protein, because protein cannot be absorbed in greater quantities than the allowed portions in one sitting!

And don't just use the above samples. Do whatever you want. But remember the following rules:

1. 2–3 portions of protein daily.
2. 4–6 portions of complex carbohydrates daily.
3. 2–4 portions of simple carbohydrates daily.
4. 3–5 cups *minimum* of unlimited free complex carbohydrates.
5. Keep fat grams 25 or below (you will get most of your fat from the protein).
6. Eat often—try for five or more times a day. Try not to go more than four hours without eating.

Free Eating Day Once a Week When You Reach Your Goal

Once you reach your goal, you can eat anything you want, all day long, once a week. And yes, this really works. By keeping to the diet guidelines all week long, you allow yourself leeway—the leeway to consume extra fat and calories one day a week. If you continued to follow the low-fat eating plan in this chapter for the rest of your life, never taking a free eating day even when you reached your ideal body, you would eventually lose too much weight and you would become too thin.

Sure. I could tell you to instead include a forbidden food once a day instead of waiting for once a week to pig out all day, but frankly, that wouldn't work for most people, because it's very difficult to cope with that much temptation—to eat one forbidden food and then go on with appropriate eating for the rest of the day. The majority of people who love to eat would rather be "a good girl," all week, and then feel that they have earned the reward of a free eating day at the end of the week.

When you first try this out, you may be inclined to call my bluff and start eating early in the morning and go straight to midnight in an effort to get in as much as you can—bacon and eggs, steak and fries, shakes and pizza, donuts, chocolate cake, ice cream, the works. Okay. Do that. You'll be as sick as a dog the next day, and the next week you won't be so crazy. In time you'll relax and just eat a few foods that you've been missing. You'll realize that those foods are not going anywhere—and if you don't get them all in on your free eating day this week, you can always do it next week.

Without the free eating day, I would probably resent my life and eventually just lose control and start eating whatever I wanted all week. But I don't have to do that because my favorite foods await me on Saturday: cream cheese, cheeze-its, Tootsie Rolls, pizza, and once in a while a juicy red steak! The beautiful part is, you never have to permanently give up your favorite goodies.

SPECIAL SEVEN-DAY DIET TO LOOK FIVE TO TEN POUNDS THINNER

In order to look five to ten pounds thinner—in a sense, in order to trick your body into looking thin and in fact being temporarily thin quickly—you can take advantage of a milder form of an extreme diet that bodybuilders use just before contests: higher protein/lower carbohydrates and sodium. If you follow this diet for a week, your body will appear lean and defined! You won't look as ripped as a bodybuilder, because you will not be taking the diet to the unhealthy extremes that bodybuilders do. You will be cutting down your carbohydrates and sodium, and increasing your protein intake, whereas bodybuilders who use this diet practically eliminate carbohydrates completely.

The diet works by causing your body to let go of all excess water. To get an idea of why this happens when you decrease sodium and carbohydrates, read pages 223–224—only realize that we are not taking it to an extreme here.

This diet is to be used for an emergency—say a vacation where you'll be seen in your bathing suit all week. If you do this, you can actually eat whatever you want to eat on vacation. It will take at least four days before your body starts to gain back the water weight. If you try to avoid high-sodium foods (that's the only thing you'll have to watch), you will look lean for the entire week.

How much sodium, carbohydrate, and protein will you consume? You won't have to count grams or milligrams. Just follow the guideline and sample meal plan below. But FYI: your sodium level will be under 1,500 per day.

Using the Diet for More Than a Week

What would happen if you tried to use the diet for the long term? You could do this for as long as three weeks and you would look even thinner and even more ripped. In such a case, be sure to not cut your sodium level until the last week. It's a waste of self-discipline. If you follow the diet for three weeks, it will take a bit more of an adjustment to return to normal fat-loss eating. I'll discuss this at the very end of the chapter.

Could you follow this diet for months at a time? Not a good idea. It is not a balanced diet and you would not be able to stay on it forever. Your body would rebel, and soon you would be looking for quick fixes of simple sugars. In addition, after the first few weeks your body will have given up all its excess water and you would stop losing water weight.

THE DIET

Breakfast

1 portion protein (1 yellow of egg, 3 egg whites, or 6 ounces white meat poultry)
½ cup unlimited complex carbohydrates (1 sliced tomato)

Snack

1 fruit (½ grapefruit, ½ cantaloupe, or 1 banana)

Lunch

1 portion protein (4–6 ounces tuna in water, flounder, sole, or 6 ounces white meat poultry)
1 portion limited complex carbohydrates (2 slices whole wheat bread, 1 potato, 1 cup corn, or ⅔ cup rice)
½–1 cup unlimited complex carbohydrates (1 large cucumber, large tomato and lettuce salad, 3 large red peppers, or 1 cup frozen vegetables)

Snack

1 cup unlimited complex carbohydrates (1 cup green beans or 1 cup peas and carrots)

Dinner

1 portion protein (6 ounces white meat chicken, turkey, or low-fat fish)
1 cup unlimited complex carbohydrates (1 cup cauliflower or 1 cup broccoli)

Snack

1 portion protein (4 ounces tuna in water or 6 ounces white meat chicken)
1 slice whole wheat bread

Rules

1. You may only choose whole wheat bread, baked potatoes, corn, or rice for your limited complex carbohydrates.
2. Use the above menu—eat only the foods listed on that menu for the entire week. You may, however, mix the meals and the foods around any way you choose.
3. Always rinse the tuna in water to get rid of excess sodium.
4. 1–2 portions of limited complex carbohydrates (only potatoes, corn, whole wheat bread, or rice).
5. 2–3 cups of unlimited complex carbohydrates (anything on the above menu until the last two days, when your choice is limited to green beans, peas, and carrots).
6. 1–2 fruits a day (grapefruit is the best choice).
7. 4–5 portions of protein (remember to rinse tuna in water). White meat poultry is lower in sodium than fish. Toward the last few days, use more poultry than fish for your protein source.
8. No dairy products except for milk in coffee.
9. When given an option for unlimited complex carbohydrates, limited complex carbohydrates, and fruits, try to choose the lesser, rather than the higher amount. On the other hand, feel free to eat the allowed extra protein.

Going Back to the Regular Low-Fat Eating Plan

Whether you've used the diet for a week or three weeks, you'll have to be careful once you go off the diet, because your body will crave high-sodium foods in order to make up for the low-sodium diet it has been following. Your body will also crave lots of carbohydrates, and if you're not careful, may try to trick you into eating fatty, sugary, quick-fix foods. If you let your body run its high-sodium course for a few days (a week if you've been on the diet for two or three weeks), and make sure to feed yourself the full six allowed limited complex carbohydrates and lots of free unlimited complex carbohydrates, you'll be back on course in a week—but in any case, you won't gain fat weight. You'll just gain back temporary water weight.

A Final Word About Dieting

Why bother with the seven-day diet in the first place? Good question. Why bother? Ideally, you should not have to. You should simply follow the regular low-fat eating plan and slowly get rid of all of your excess fat, while at the same time following the Definition workout. In this way you will eventually look lean and defined without ever having to use the emergency diet.

But what if you are not there yet and want to look good now? Well, I thought I'd give you a little secret that you could use—as long as you realize it is not a solution, but a device used for a purpose—a temporary diet to help you to make a good showing in an emergency. And we all know that these emergencies do come up!

The most important thing to me is that you don't misunderstand and start using that diet all the time. If you do so, you will defeat your purpose. In the long run, you won't lose as much fat and weight as you would if you followed the regular low-fat, high-carbohydrate diet in this chapter. If you use it only for a week to three weeks, say once or twice a year, it won't hinder your fat loss and no harm will be done. Case closed.

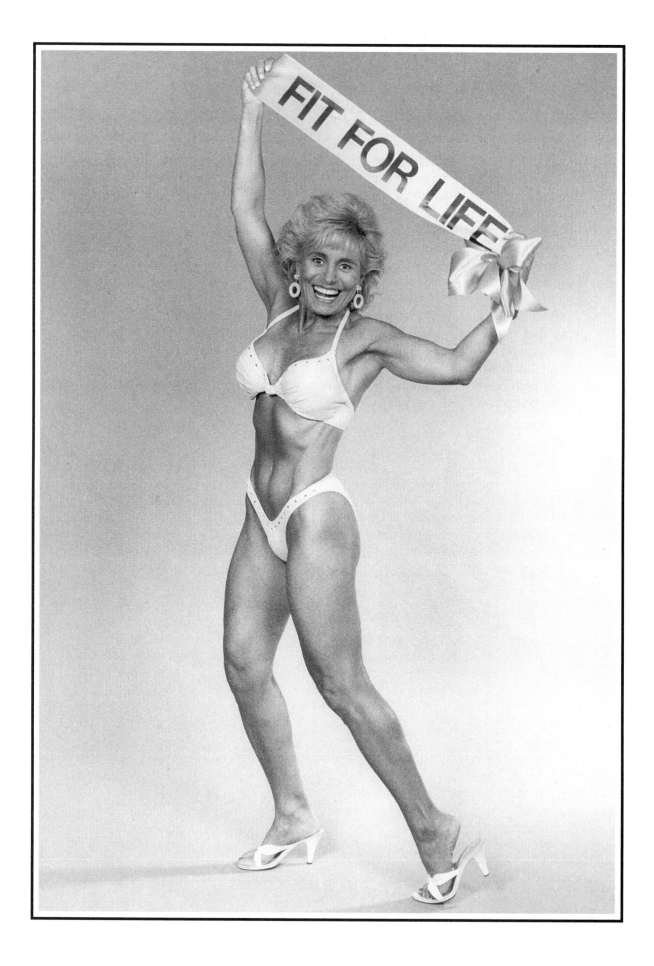

10

HOW TO MAINTAIN YOUR SHAPE FOR THE REST OF YOUR LIFE!

Do I have to do this for the rest of my life?" This is the most common question I get from people who are ready to start one of my workout plans. Not yet hooked on feeling and looking good, I suppose they are worried that the workout will one day become boring—and they are right, it probably would after a few years.

The answer is no. You don't have to do *this* workout for the rest of your life; in fact, you shouldn't! The ideal system is to switch to a different one of my workouts from time to time, according to the way your body is developing, and also to meet your current time schedule as well as your evolving psychological needs. In fact, it is very important that you tune in to your prevailing circumstances and make the timely switch in order to guarantee that your body does not become too comfortable with the routine and stop making progress—and also, in order that your mind does not become so bored with the routine that you end up merely going through the motions (and worse, going through half motions).

The longest you should do any one of my routines before switching (you can of course go back to it after a while) is about two years. The shortest time to give a routine is about six months (I'll explain the exceptions later).

Let's talk about each of my workouts. I'll point out the strongest point of the workout, and focus on why you should do it, and when. I'll start with my least muscle-building, and shortest workout, the 12-Minute Total-Body Workout, and end with my most muscle-building and longest workout, Now or Never. In between you'll find Definition, the Fat-Burning Workout and Bottoms Up! Each workout has its own special features. For example, each workout utilizes a different workout principle and challenges your muscles in a unique way—so that if you make timely switches, over a lifetime, your muscles are challenged in every possible way. In addition, each workout includes some common basic exercises, but features exercises not in any other book.

WHY CHANGE WORKOUTS FROM TIME TO TIME?

The reason for changing your workout every so often has to do with the time-tested principle of muscle confusion. To prevent fatigue of mind and body, most champion bodybuilders change their routine periodically, "confusing" the muscles and, in effect, not allowing them to become complacent, thinking they "know the routine" and not working as hard. Some people take this to an extreme, and change their routines almost every time they work out. This can only be done, however, if you are seasoned in working out and know what you're doing. When you get to that point, you can mix and match my workouts within a given week. I'll discuss this at the end of the chapter.

THE 12-MINUTE TOTAL-BODY WORKOUT

This is an excellent workout for those who are complete *beginners* and who have very little time to invest in working out, or who are not completely sold on working with weights and need to be convinced before they make a bigger time commitment. It is also the perfect workout to do when *traveling* (you can do it with no weights, or you can get water weights for traveling) no matter what your regular workout regimen is.

It is also the perfect workout to do if you have an *injury* you have to work around, because you use very light weights. (Of course you would show this book to your doctor and let him help you choose the exercises you can safely perform.) In addition, it is the ideal workout to switch to if you are *burned out* from your regular workout and would like an easier change of pace. Finally, it is the perfect workout for those in their seventh through ninth months of *pregnancy*—only with the doctor's permission of course—and for the first three weeks after the baby is born.

The strongest feature of this workout is its ability to produce muscle hardness! As the name indicates, the workout takes only twelve minutes. The only equipment you need is a set of three-pound dumbbells (three pounds each). You do this workout every single day, so it is wonderful for establishing a habit that you will eventually blindly do—like brushing your teeth every morning.

This workout does not increase muscle size at all, unless you have very underdeveloped muscles. It tightens and tones existing muscles—in short, it makes your entire body harder.

The workout is also extremely simple to perform. You do all three sets of every exercise with three-pound dumbbells and ten repetitions. (In other words, you do not use the pyramid system.) The workout principle that dominates this workout is dynamic tension, or isometric pressure. In other words, you continually put pressure on the working muscle—you continually flex and tense the muscle from the start of the movement until the finish.

I learned this technique by a combination of my knowledge of bodybuilding techniques and methods of martial artists. By moving the weights in the same manner as bodybuilders—and squeezing your muscles as hard as possible, the way marital artists do when they perform their kata (the dancelike practice of punching and blocking movements), you tighten your flabby muscles until they are as hard as a rock.

In the past, I said that you can get maximum definition with this workout, but I have since learned that this is not the case. You do get some definition, but the major force of this workout is to harden your muscles. Some definition is a secondary factor.

You don't need any equipment for this workout other than the three-pound dumbbells, and in fact, once you are used to the workout with the dumbbells, you can do it without any weights (you will have learned by then to completely create your own force by applying constant pressure). Since you are using such light (or no) weights for the workout, you won't even need a bench. You can do the exercises that normally require a bench by tipping a chair back or placing your back on the edge of a bed or sofa.

I do this workout for weeks at a time when I'm on the road, or when I am burned out and need a rest from working out, but don't want to completely stop working out (except for a planned week, I never completely stop working out).

This workout can keep your body in shape for months at a time. The proof is, say for example you are used to doing a much more strenuous workout, and then you switch to this workout for a month. When you go back to your regular workout, you won't feel excessive aches and pains the next day. In fact, you may not feel any aches or pains, whereas had you stopped working out completely for a month, the day after you started working out with your regular routine again, you would be so sore that you would hardly be able to move.

Why is it that such a seemingly insignificant workout can have such a powerful effect? The answer is simple. The 12-Minute Total-Body Workout challenges all nine body parts in such an intense way that every muscle fiber participates in the movement. In turn, your muscles never get the chance to go to sleep, and when you resume your regular workout—even though you may be using heavier weights, and working for a longer period of time—your muscles are ready to go because they have been asked to flex and use tension to the maximum.

In addition to everything else, doing the 12-Minute Total-Body Workout teaches you the discipline of maximum flexing and continual application of tension to the working muscle, and this discipline carries over to any workout you do. Even when you increase your weights as in my other workouts, it's still a good idea to flex and apply pressure to the maximum of your ability (although of course, due to increased use of weight, you will not be able to apply the same degree of flexing and continual pressure).

DEFINITION

This is an excellent workout for beginners who are looking for a workout that will give them both a complete aerobic workout, and at the same time, a total-body workout that will add a small amount of muscle size and maximum definition. In addition, it is great for those who want to be able to work out only three days a week (because it is my only workout that allows you to exercise the entire body in one day and still get the maximum out of the workout).

It is also an ideal workout for those who have been working out for a while with any of my other workouts, but who want to get more definition—because *the strongest feature of this workout is, as the title indicates, its ability to give maximum definition in a super-fat-burning aerobic weight-training routine.*

This workout is also great for people who have been working with any of my longer workouts, and want a slightly shorter one (fifteen minutes, six days a week, or thirty minutes, three days a week) that burns maximum fat yet continues to build some muscle, although not as much muscle as the longer workout.

This is also the workout for those who are hooked on aerobics, and who want to feel as if they are doing an aerobic workout, even though they are working with weights.

The workout principle that dominates this workout is the full pyramid system (it is my only book that utilizes the full pyramid system) combined with the speed superset! I won't explain them here, since you already know them, having read this book.

THE FAT-BURNING WORKOUT

This workout is ideal for those who want to put on a little more muscle than you can with Definition, but still burn maximum fat, and for those who have a little more time to invest (twenty minutes, four to six days a week).

The workout uses the giant-set principle—you challenge a given body part to the extreme—and in turn, get a great deal of definition (but not quite as much as in Definition, yet a little more than in Bottoms Up!).

You do your first set of all three exercises for a given body part before you rest, raise your weight, and do your second set of all three exercises for that body part, and so on. In short, it is very similar to Definition, only you don't go down the pyramid—you do the modified pyramid system. The Fat-Burning Workout requires that you do only three sets before you rest—your first set of three exercises; but Definition requires that you do ten sets before you rest— your first five supersets of two exercises for a body part. This can be a welcome change for your muscles. It allows more growth and does not exhaust the muscles as much as Definition does.

The strongest point of the Fat-Burning Workout is, you can get significant muscular development and, at the same time, burn a great deal of fat. In order to save workout time, in Definition I have eliminated all exercises that require working one arm or leg at a time, so the Fat-Burning Workout has many exercises not found in Definition.

Even if you are crazy about Definition, it is a good idea to switch to the Fat-Burning Workout after about six months to a year, two at the most, if for no other reason than to challenge the muscles with different exercises that can hit them from various angles, and in addition, to get more muscular development.

The Fat-Burning Workout requires the use of three sets of dumbbells: three pounds, five pounds, and ten pounds, but those who are beginners often find that they must go as low as one-, two-, and three-pound dumbbells, especially if they are using my accompanying video (see Bibliography), which requires that they keep up a very fast pace. If you do start with very light weights, you can of course eventually work your way up to the higher weights.

BOTTOMS UP!

This workout is excellent for those women who need extra work for the lower and middle body, and want the option of doing the minimum or maximum amount of work for the upper body. For example, Bottoms Up! requires that you do seven exercises each for hips/buttocks and thighs, while the Fat-Burning Workout requires only three exercises for those body parts—and offers an option of two more. In addition, Bottoms Up! offers special work for the inner thigh and the saddlebags, and gives a mandatory bombs-away stomach routine.

The workout uses the principles of the modified pyramid system, in combination with the twin set. Instead of exhausting one body part before moving to the next body part (as you do in the Fat-Burning Workout and in Definition), Bottoms Up! allows you to alternately exercise two body parts at a time, so that while one body part is working, the other body part is resting, and so that you never have to stop and take a rest—and hence, can burn more fat than ever. (If you don't take your optional rests, this workout is completely aerobic.)

For example, with Bottoms Up! you do one set of a thigh exercise, say, the squat, and without resting, one set of a butt exercise, say, the back leg kick. Then, because your thighs have rested while you were doing the butt exercise, you can go right back and do your second set of your thigh exercise, and so on, until you complete all seven sets of the combined exercises.

The beauty of this system is, you no longer dread exercising your thighs, because the difficulty and the tedium are gone. The same principle holds true when working any other body part, because all body parts are paired into twins. You exercise the chest in combination with the shoulders, the biceps in combination with the triceps, and so on.

Bottoms Up! is ideal for those who feel too much muscle fatigue when doing Definition or the Fat-Burning Workout, because it does not place as great a demand on a given muscle (due to the alternate exercises—the switching back and forth from an exercise for one body part, say, thighs, to another body part, say, buttocks, which allows one muscle to rest while the other muscle is working).

The strongest point of Bottoms Up! is that it allows you to build more muscle than do the 12-Minute Total-Body Workout, Definition, or the Fat-Burning Workout, and that it gives extra work for the hips, buttocks, thighs, and abdominals. On the other hand, it gives a good deal of definition, but not as much definition as you get with the Fat-Burning Workout, and not nearly as much as you get with the Definition workout. You need three sets of dumbbells: three pounds, five pounds, and eight pounds, and as in all of my workouts except the 12-Minute Total-Body Workout, you must raise your weights when they become too easy to lift. You do Bottoms Up! four to six days a week, and the workout takes twenty to thirty minutes, depending upon whether or not you take the optional rests allowed after each twin set.

NOW OR NEVER

This is my most traditional workout. It takes about an hour to do because you are working with heavier weights, and must rest about thirty seconds between each set. It is the ideal workout for those who want to put on significant muscle size, or for those who want to add muscle to a given body part. For example, you can do this workout for only the body part you want to increase. For instance, you may want to use the Now or Never thigh workout if you want to add muscle to your front thigh so that the skin no longer sags over your knee!

Now or Never has an illustrated machine workout, so if you want to go to a fitness center, and if you like incorporating machines into your workout, you may want to try this book. Even if you don't want to use the Now or Never routine, if you get a copy of the book, you can use it to illustrate the machine alternatives (I do not illustrate them in my other books, except in Top Shape (see below), I just tell you which machine alternatives to use).

Now or Never is the ideal workout to begin with to establish a muscle base. This would be great if you were already committed and determined, had the time (an hour per workout), and if you were not afraid of muscles. I find that most people need to be coaxed into the fuller commitment of Now or Never by first experimenting with my other workouts. Then, once they see that muscle making is not a matter of picking up a weight and the next day blowing up into a female Arnold, but that in fact, muscle is hard to earn, and comes slowly, over time, they are not afraid to do a workout such as is found in Now or Never. I started out with Now or Never for about a year, invented and switched to the 12-Minute Total-Body Workout for a year, invented and switched to the Fat-Burning Workout for a year and a half, invented and switched to Bottoms Up! for a year and a half, and invented and switched to Definition for a year. In between, I did Top Shape and added in Gut Busters from time to time—while I was inventing those workouts.

You will know if it is time to switch to Now or Never. The simple rule of thumb will be: do you want more muscular development than you are getting with my other workouts? If you do want more muscular development, switch to Now or Never for six months to two years, and then switch to either the Fat-Burning Workout or Definition for a dramatic change and maximum definition, or to Bottoms Up! for a less dramatic change and some added definition.

Now or Never utilizes the modified pyramid system. *Its strongest point is its capacity for maximum muscle building.* Since you must rest thirty seconds between each set (you may choose to rest only fifteen seconds) this is not considered to be an aerobic workout. (You can of course do the extra aerobics suggested in the book.) But keep in mind, since you build the maximum muscle with this workout, it gives you the permanent ability to burn more fat twenty-four hours a day, since muscle raises your resting metabolism (see pages 3–4).

You do the Now or Never workout four to six days a week. You start out using three-, five-, and ten-pound dumbbells with this workout, but you continually advance, until you are eventually using ten, fifteen, and twenty pounds—or higher, depending upon which body part you are exercising, and how much muscle you want to add to your body.

Remember that all of the workouts build muscle (except for the 12-Minute Total-Body Workout, which hardens the muscle you already have). It is the degree we are talking about here. Also keep in mind that all of my workout books provide a total-body workout.

WHEN TO SWITCH

It is ideal to give any workout six months before thinking of switching to a new workout. If you really want to see what the workout can do for you, give it an entire year. Then if you like what you're seeing, give it another six months. Then evaluate. If you still like what you're seeing, stick with it for another six months. Then, no matter what, you should switch.

DECIDING WHAT TO SWITCH TO

Let's start with the assumption that you have been doing Definition for six months to a year. What you switch to will depend upon what you see in the mirror, and how you now feel about working out. Assuming you are willing to put in just a little more time: if when you look in the mirror, you see lots of definition, but not enough overall muscular development for your liking, you can switch either to Now or Never or to Bottoms Up!

If when you look in the mirror, you see lots of definition, but you notice that your lower and middle body need more work, switch to Bottoms Up! If you love Definition, but are ready for a change, and you want to challenge the muscles from different angles, yet continue to have a maximum fat-burning workout, but one that allows slightly more muscular development, switch to the Fat-Burning Workout—it is the most similar to Definition, yet is not quite as exhausting. It utilizes a different workout system—the giant set, so that your muscles will be challenged in a new way.

If you're getting burned out from working out and your muscles are screaming at you for a break, switch to the 12-Minute Total-Body Workout. Instead of fifteen minutes, six days a week, you'll be working out twelve minutes every day—but with a wonderfully opposite workout. Instead of working your muscles in an aerobic way to complete exhaustion, your muscles will be asked to continually flex and tense. You'll be allowed more rests. Your muscles will welcome the change by responding with increased hardness and density.

Suppose you've been doing the Fat-Burning Workout, and you love that workout, but would like to get even more definition. Switch to Definition—it's very similar, and in some ways, even more challenging, because you are going up and down the pyramid—doing the full pyramid system instead of the modified pyramid.

Suppose you've been doing the Fat-Burning Workout, but your muscles are becoming fatigued—and you would also like to get a slight bit more muscle size. Switch to Bottoms Up! That workout utilizes the twin set, which allows one muscle to rest while the other is working. It's not as exhausting, and in the bargain, you'll get extra work for your middle and lower body, and you'll burn as much or more fat as in the Fat-Burning Workout. Suppose you are doing the Fat-Burning Workout, but realize that you want to take time out to build a bigger muscle base. Switch to Now or Never.

Suppose you are doing Bottoms Up! and are tired of that routine and want to challenge your muscles to exhaustion and at the same time get more definition—and yet continue to build muscle. Try the Fat-Burning Workout. Suppose you've been doing Bottoms Up! and want the maximum amount of definition, and you want to build a very small amount of muscle—and in the bargain, you want to be able to get the workout over with in only three workout days a week. Switch to Definition!

Suppose you are doing Bottoms Up! and are excited about the muscles you are getting, but want even bigger muscles: switch to Now or Never.

What if you are doing the 12-Minute Total-Body Workout, and you want to burn maximum fat and get maximum definition—but still keep the workout short? Switch to Definition. What if you are doing the 12-Minute Total-Body Workout, and you need more work for your lower and middle body, but are happy with your upper body the way it is? Switch to Bottoms Up! for the lower body only, and continue doing the 12-Minute Total-Body Workout for the upper body. What if you're doing the 12-Minute Total-Body Workout and you want to put on a stronger muscle base? Switch to Now or Never.

WHAT IF YOU DON'T KNOW WHAT YOU'RE DOING— CAN YOU JUST SWITCH AT RANDOM?

Good news. Yes. Even if you put the names of my books in a basket, and picked one out at random, and did if for six months, and then switched at random to another for six months, and so on, you would have your equivalent of the body you see on the cover of this book—and better. This is a promise.

Why would this work? By switching back and forth, even at random, you would be utilizing the basic body-shaping techniques perfected over time by champion bodybuilders—techniques that, in a scientific manner, shape and define the body into its most symmetrical form—and you would be taking advantage of the time-tested principle of muscle confusion.

But you don't have to rely on random choice. In fact, you can choose which workout to do based upon the above guidelines, and your specific needs at a given time in your life. The point is, you need never get out of shape, because you need never stop working out.

In review, here is the list of my exercise books according to length of workout, from shortest to longest—from least muscle-building to most muscle-building.

1. *The 12-Minute Total-Body Workout*—twelve minutes every day.
2. *Definition*—fifteen minutes, six days a week or thirty minutes, three days a week.
3. *The Fat-Burning Workout*—twenty minutes, four to six days a week.
4. *Bottoms Up!*—thirty minutes, four to six days a week (if you take no rests, twenty minutes).
5. *Now or Never*—sixty to ninety minutes, four to six days a week (if you shorten the rests, forty minutes).

AND SPEAKING OF TIME

You must realize that the stated time is based upon the assumption that you are used to the workout. In the beginning, all of the workouts take much longer. In addition, the above calculations are based upon the assumption that you are doing the regular workout.

You always have the option of doing the extra work—such as the *Wonder Woman* and *Dragon Lady* workouts in Definition, the *Intensity* and *Insanity* workouts in the Fat-Burning Workout, and the *Wild Woman* and *Terminator* workouts in Bottoms Up! These plans add ten to twenty minutes per workout.

WHAT ABOUT GUT BUSTERS AND TOP SHAPE?

You may have noticed that I have two books that feature men on the cover. Can women do these workouts? Absolutely yes. In fact, I do Gut Busters on alternate days for my stomach (from time to time). If you have a really "problem" stomach, I suggest that you do Gut Busters on the days you don't do your stomach for your regular workout.

What about *Top Shape*? Top Shape is a similar workout to Now or Never, but with different exercises, and it is a shorter workout. It's an excellent book to switch to if you are doing Now or Never and want to continue to build muscle, but are getting bored with the exercises. Beware of one thing however: there are no hips/buttocks exercises in *Top Shape*, because men do not have childbearing hips, and do not need work in that area, so if you switch to that book, continue to do your hips/butt exercises from any of my other books, perhaps from *Bottoms Up!* In addition, you will notice that the leg workout is optional in *Top Shape*. For women, the leg workout is not optional, so do the leg workout in that book!

Top Shape also has an illustrated machine workout, so even if you are not going to use this book, you can refer to the photographs and use them for the gym alternatives in any of my other books (where I tell you the alternatives, but do not include photographs of the exercises).

WHERE DOES THE COLLEGE DORM WORKOUT FIT IN?

This workout was invented by my daughter, Marthe Simone. She took all of my workouts and created one that can be done in twenty minutes with only five-pound dumbbells in a small space—with virtually no other equipment. It is a mini Fat-Burning Workout with overtones of the 12-Minute Total-Body Workout! You can switch to this if you are tired of doing the 12-Minute Total-Body Workout and want a bit more of a challenge and yet not quite as much of a challenge as the Fat-Burning Workout or one of the other books. This book also has an eating plan that will help you to deal with the most impossible menus.

MIXING AND MATCHING WORKOUTS

Yes. You can decide to do, say, Bottoms Up! for the lower and middle body only, and the Fat-Burning Workout, Now or Never, Definition, or the 12-Minute Total-Body Workout for the upper body. Another example: you can do the Fat-Burning Workout for all body parts except biceps and triceps—and use Now or Never for those body parts, because you may want to put more muscle in your arms so that they no longer wave like flags. You may decide to do the 12-Minute Total-Body Workout for everything except the stomach—and instead do Gut Busters every day for the stomach. You may decide to do Definition for the upper body only, Gut Busters for the middle body, and Bottoms Up! for the lower body.

Once you get a feeling for what working out is all about, you can be creative and mix and match the workouts according to your needs. But don't feel as if you're obligated to do that. Even if you stick to one complete workout at a time you will eventually create a near-perfect body.

SWITCHING FROM ONE WORKOUT TO ANOTHER IN A GIVEN WEEK

Now this really takes confidence and creativity. I'm a creature of habit, so I would never do this—I need a humdrum steady routine. But if you are more adventurous, once you know what you're doing—say for example you've used two of my workouts already, and are quite familiar with working out—you can use the workout from one book on one day, and another book on another day. As long as you remember to not work the same body parts two days in a row (except for abdominals, which can be exercised every day), you will be fine.

For example, you may decide that you want to do Now or Never for the lower body on Monday, and the Fat-Burning Workout for the upper body on Tuesday, and back to Now or Never for the lower body on Wednesday, and back to the Fat-Burning Workout for the upper body on Thursday, and so on; and in the bargain, do Gut Busters every day for the stomach, instead of the stomach workout in either Now or Never or the Fat-Burning Workout.

Or you may want to do Bottoms Up! on Monday for the lower and middle body, and Definition for the upper body on Tuesday, and so on, switching back and forth.

You can even go a step further and do as many as four workouts in a given week. For example, you can do Definition for the upper body on Monday, the Fat-Burning Workout for the lower and middle body on Tuesday, Now or Never for the upper body on Wednesday, and Bottoms Up! for the lower and middle body on Thursday. In fact, this is an excellent plan because it keeps the body challenged in every possible way. It is probably the most ideal way to work out. As mentioned above, I am a creature of habit and don't do it myself, but other people I know do, and their bodies look even better than mine. Someday I plan to force myself to try it. I'll wait until I really need a challenge.

There's no limit to what you can do. If you are confident, and are not afraid of confusing yourself, go for it. If you are in doubt of what you are doing, write to me and I'll confirm or disavow it—but please include a photograph of yourself so I can give an intelligent opinion (also be sure to include a stamped, self-addressed envelope).

HOW TO STAY IN SHAPE FOR THE REST OF YOUR LIFE—
EVEN IF YOU GO HOG WILD WITH YOUR DIET!

My secret for staying in shape is, even if I go to complete abandonment with my diet—if I pig out for weeks at a time, or even months at a time—*I never stop working out.*

No one can be perfect all the time. We all need to let down our guard from time to time. I love to eat, and look forward to weeks or even a couple of months of eating whatever I please. When I do this, I slowly gain fat weight—about a half a pound to a pound a week, until I gain about five to six pounds. When I reach my highest weight, about 123, I begin to eat right again, and I slowly lose the weight.

But why is it that even while I was pigging out for weeks, I didn't also stop working out? After all, if I were going to let myself go, I might as well go all the way, right? Wrong. In fact, that would be the worst mistake I could make. I continue to do the workout, so that my muscles will still be there, under the fat, and so that when I begin to eat right again, all I have to do is wait for the extra layer or two of fat to melt away—and reveal the already existing muscles. In addition, if I had stopped working out for those weeks, my metabolism (my ability to burn fat twenty-four hours a day) would have decreased, because when muscle decreases, metabolism goes down (see page 3 for a review of this principle), and I would have gotten even fatter.

There's another reason to never stop working out—even though you are completely ignoring good eating habits. It helps keep your overeating in check—to a certain extent. You see, even if you are bound and determined to eat like a pig, if you're still working out, your body will actually stop you from going too far because the workout will stimulate your healthy muscles and bones, and circulating blood, to cry out to you and pull you toward eating foods that nourish and energize them—such as low-fat protein and carbohydrates, and fruits and vegetables. In spite of yourself, you will find yourself eating these foods in the midst of your determination to eat only junk—if and only if you don't stop working out.

On the other hand, if you stop working out, and concurrently pig out for weeks at a time, your body will get into a rut. It will become mesmerized. It will not cry out as quickly for better eating habits—your muscles, bones, and blood will become sluggish—almost hypnotized. In addition, your mind will not be as alert to your body. Your mind will ignore your body's pleas for a better diet. It may take six months before your body realizes what you are doing to it, and by that time you will have gained back so much weight, and lost some muscle, that it will feel as if you are starting from scratch.

So if you're going to go hog wild, no matter what you do, don't go all the way and abandon both your workout and your good eating habits. Let the good eating habits go for a short time but keep working out, unless, of course, you have medical problems.

There is also another catch. Even if you want to do this, you can't do it until you have achieved your ideal body and held it for about a year. Then you are in at least some control. Let me explain how this works.

Before you can dare let yourself experiment with this method, you have to make sure that your body has had time to experience the feeling of being at its ideal fitness level. This way your body will have a point of reference—a sense of where you *ought* to be when you go off base. If you try to let go of good eating habits before you've achieved your ideal fitness level in the first place, your body will have no sense of what is right—what is ideal—and when you pig out day after day, your body will slip back to where you were when you first started. In other words, you need to set up a base so that a momentum can be created to pull you back there (your ideal fitness level) before this system can work for you.

I'm not recommending that you try this method. In fact, I would rather see you maintain good eating habits all year round once you get in shape—taking advantage of only the one-day-a-week free eating day. Many of the women who write to me do just that. But in case you're like me, I wanted to share with you my secret. I am a pig at heart. No—not a pig, a dog. In fact, I often wish I had a long snout like a dog so I could put my face in the plate and eat even faster—the way dogs do. I love to eat, and I always will love to eat. I also hate rules and regimens that can't ever be broken. So when I find a way to be able to break the rules within reason, I do it.

One final note. Why can't you do the reverse when you want to go to hell with yourself—stop working out but maintain good eating habits? You can do that, but you will slowly lose muscle—and you won't enjoy eating while you're doing it. That's no fun at all! In addition to losing muscle, your body will begin to feel soft. You won't feel sexy. Your energy level will decrease, your posture will begin to return to its old slump, and you'll lose definition. You won't feel as strong, and your self-esteem will slowly decrease. Whereas if you kept working out, none of the above would happen—except that you might feel a little guilty about overeating (and this is good—it reminds you that you must soon get back to good eating habits).

CAN YOU EVER TAKE TIME OFF FROM WORKING OUT?

Yes. Of course you can. You can take a week off, and in an extreme case, ten days every six months. It's never a good idea to willfully take off more time than that—and there's absolutely no excuse for it. No matter where you are in the world, you can always do a workout—even with no weights and no equipment (for example, you can do the 12-Minute Total-Body Workout).

If you find yourself getting burned out, you can take a week off as often as every six months. In fact, once a year, just to prevent burnout, you should take a week off from working out with weights. You can walk, play sports, and/or do some favorite aerobic activity, but take time off from the weights.

Should you take a week off and completely stagnate? I don't recommend it. You can let your body do what it pleases for a week, but I have a feeling that your body won't just want to stagnate. Even on a vacation, your body will enjoy swimming, engaging in sports, and walking around. If you try to just vegetate, your body will not be happy. By the end of the week you'll feel sluggish. You won't enjoy your vacation as much. So follow your "body voice," and just enjoy yourself for a week, but don't punish your body by refusing to let it move if it asks to move. You know what I'm talking about.

A FINAL WORD

You've read the book, but you may have a question. If you do, I'll be happy to answer you, but I cannot answer unless you send a stamped, self-addressed envelope.

Joyce L. Vedral
P.O. Box 7433-0433
Wantagh, NY 11793-0433

To Order Cast-Iron Dumbbells—Shipping Included

A set of one-, two-, and three-pound dumbbells needed for this workout, $34.99 (*not sold separately*).

Set of five-pound dumbbells, $23.00
Set of eight-pound dumbbells, $33.00
Set of ten-pound dumbbells, $40.00
Set of twelve-pound dumbbells, $47.00
Set of fifteen-pound dumbbells, $55.00

Note: Shipping dumbbells is expensive. Check your local gym equipment stores and save money by purchasing them direct from the stores. I offer this as a service for those who cannot find dumbbells, or who want the convenience of ordering them.

Color Photo (8"×10") Autographed to You by Me! $12.00.

All of the above items are shipped UPS, prepaid.

Three- or Five-Pound Water Weights

Call 1-800-251-6040 to order.

For videos, see pages 259–260.

BIBLIOGRAPHY

BOOKS BY JOYCE VEDRAL

Vedral, Joyce, Ph.D. *Top Shape*. New York: Warner Books, 1995.

Vedral, Marthe S., and Joyce L. Vedral. *The College Dorm Workout*. New York: Warner Books, 1994.

Vedral, Joyce, Ph.D. *Bottoms Up!* New York: Warner Books, 1993.

Vedral, Joyce, Ph.D. *Gut Busters*. New York: Warner Books, 1992.

Vedral, Joyce, Ph.D. *The Fat-Burning Workout*. New York: Warner Books, 1991.

Vedral, Joyce, Ph.D. *The 12-Minute Total-Body Workout*. New York: Warner Books, 1989.

Vedral, Joyce, Ph.D. *Now or Never*. New York: Warner Books, 1986.

Vedral, Joyce, Ph.D. *Get Rid of Him*. New York: Warner Books, 1993.

VIDEOS BY JOYCE VEDRAL

Vedral, Joyce, Ph.D. *The Bottoms Up Workout: Upper Body*, Good Times Video, 1995, New York. (All video stores, or call 1-800-433-6769 or 612-571-5840.)

Vedral, Joyce, Ph.D. *The Bottoms Up Workout: Middle Body*, Good Times Video, 1995, New York. (All video stores, or call 1-800-433-6769 or 612-571-5840.)
Vedral, Joyce, Ph.D. *The Bottoms Up Workout: Lower Body*, Good Times Video, 1995, New York. (All video stores, or call 1-800-433-6769 or 612-571-5840.)
Vedral, Joyce, Ph.D. *The Fat-Burning Workout: Volume I. The Regular Workout.* Time-Life Video, 1993, New York. (Send a check for $24.98 to Joyce Vedral, P.O. Box 7433, Wantagh, NY 11793-0433.)
Vedral, Joyce, Ph.D. *The Fat-Burning Workout: Volume II. The Intensity and Insanity Workouts.* Time-Life Video, 1993, New York. (Send a check for $24.98 to Joyce Vedral, P.O. Box 7433, Wantagh, NY 11793-0433.)

NUTRITION, DIET AND COOKBOOKS

Granader, Sherry, with foreword by Lou Ferrigno. *The Eat Right, Feel Good, Lose Weight, Have Fun Cookbook.* Houston: Larksdale Press, 1992. (Profits go to Camp-Make-A-Dream, the Children's Oncology Foundation.)
Katahn, Martin, Ph.D., and Jamie Pope Cordle, M.D., *The T-Factor Fat Gram Counter.* New York: W.W. Norton & Company.
Kirshbaum, John (ed). *The Nutrition Almanac.* New York: McGraw-Hill, 1989.
Mycoskie, Pam. *Butter Busters: The Cookbook.* New York: Warner Books, 1992.
Reynolds, Bill, and Joyce L. Vedral, Ph.D. *Supercut: Nutrition for the Ultimate Physique.* Chicago: Contemporary Books, 1987.

INDEX

ABOUT THE AUTHOR

We'll never forget the day in 1991 when Joyce Vedral appeared on the *Sally Jessy Raphaël* show. It was a quiet July morning and Joyce had been invited on the program to promote her new book, *The Fat-Burning Workout*. With a built-in flair for the dramatic, Joyce decided to appear on camera in a provocative gold bikini that showed off her toned, enviable forty-eight-year-old figure to best effect.

If we told you that all hell broke loose a mere five minutes into the broadcast, it wouldn't begin to describe the pandemonium that followed as viewers all over the country raced out to find copies of Joyce's workout. "If she can do it, I can do it too," they cried to bookstore owners, the Warner switchboard, and to anyone who would listen. In no time, Joyce was a recognized fitness guru, well on her way to the *New York Times* best-seller list.

If anyone ever tells you that lightning does not strike twice, don't believe them. Joyce did it again. Recently, she appeared on the *Montel Williams* show and had an even greater reaction to her latest book, *Bottoms Up!* For the week of January 1, 1994, her book beat all books in print in America, including Howard Stern's, Rush Limbaugh's, and Michael Crichton's—making number one on the *USA Today* list for that week.

Today, at a fit and classy fifty-two, Joyce's fitness library combines for an in-print total of well over one million copies. The reason books like *Now or Never*, *Top Shape*, *Gut Busters*, *The 12-Minute Total-Body Workout*, *Bottoms Up!*, and *The College Dorm Workout* (written with her daughter, Marthe) have sold so well is simple: they achieve the promised results.

But there's another reason for Joyce's success: Joyce, with her trademark upbeat voice, is a real person who convinces people in lectures and on television shows all over the country that "If I can do it, so can you." She isn't shy about the "before" picture of herself, fat at twenty-five, nor is she afraid to poke fun at her "bad genetics." "I come from a Russian heritage," she says. "My whole family look like boxes on wheels."

When Joyce gives a lecture, people are mesmerized. She has a way of relating to an audience as if she knows each and every one personally, and a gift for getting right down to the level of each eager listener. In the words of Paul Adamo of The Learning Annex in New York City, "In all the years of my having lecturers, I have never seen anything like this in my life. She arrests the audience and keeps each and every one of them in the palm of her hand throughout. People walk away with love in their eyes. No one can have a Joyce Vedral 'experience' without being touched."

Joyce is a frequent guest on *Oprah*, *Donahue*, *Sally Jessy Raphaël*, *Montel Williams*, *Geraldo*, and CNN, and has been written up in the *New York Times*, the *New York Daily News*, and the *New York Post*. She is a sought-after speaker in women's groups, fitness centers, and shopping malls across the country.

Perhaps what makes Joyce most interesting is her unusual background. Unlike so many other fitness experts who are one-dimensional, Joyce earned her Ph.D. in English literature with a specialization in psychology from New York University. Her knowledge of fitness came after years of teaching high school and college English, getting "fat and out of shape," and by luck landing freelance assignments to *Muscle and Fitness* and *Shape* magazines, where she became acquainted with the techniques that now fill her books and lectures. "I have a life—I'm a mother [Joyce has a twenty-three-year-old daughter], and a college professor. I don't have time to spend all day working out. I had to figure out how to fit fifteen to thirty minutes a day into my schedule and get fitness out of the way—so I could live my life in the real world. Being out of shape was draining my energy and stealing my creativity," Joyce says. "My mission is to help others who lead busy lives and are interested in getting healthy and in shape in minutes rather than hours a day."

Always a women's advocate, Joyce is in addition the author of the Warner Books international best-seller *Get Rid of Him*, a book that helps women build their self-esteem, discover their inner strength, and to move on when it's time—and to find the right man!